MULTIPLE SCLEROSIS: A NEW JOURNEY

RICHARD C. SENELICK, MD

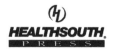

HEALTHSOUTH.
P R E S S

This book is not intended to replace personal medical care and/or professional supervision; there is no substitute for the experience and information that your doctor or health professional can provide. Rather, it is our hope that this book will provide additional information to help people understand the nature of multiple sclerosis, as well as its effects on the people with MS, their families, friends, co-workers, and the public at large. Its goal is to help people with MS live healthier and happier lives.

Proper treatment should always be tailored to the individual. If you read something in this book that seems to conflict with any of your doctors' or healthcare professionals' instructions, contact them. There may be sound reasons for recommending behavior that may differ from the information presented in this book.

If you have any questions about any treatment in this book, please consult your doctor or healthcare professional.

Also, the names and cases used in this book do not represent actual people, but are composite cases drawn from several sources.

© 2003 by HealthSouth Press
One HealthSouth Parkway, Birmingham, Alabama 35243

Published by HealthSouth Press

Library of Congress Catalog Card Number: 2002107063
ISBN: 1-891525-12-3
Second HealthSouth Printing
10 9 8 7 6 5 4 3 2
HealthSouth Press and colophon are registered
trademarks of HealthSouth
Printed in Canada

This book is dedicated to people everywhere who have MS. May they and their loved ones enjoy healthier, happier lives.

THE FACTS ABOUT HEALTHSOUTH

HealthSouth Corporation is the nation's largest physical rehabilitation healthcare provider with over 100,000 patients being treated in its facilities every day.

The HealthSouth network includes rehabilitation hospitals and acute-care medical centers, as well as outpatient rehabilitation, ambulatory surgery, and diagnostic imaging centers. Some of its diverse services include the treatment of brain injury, sports injuries, spinal cord injury, stroke, pain management, and such diagnostic services as mammography, magnetic resonance imaging (MRI), nuclear medicine, and ultrasound.

HealthSouth Press has been created to help patients and their families understand the ramifications of their injury or illness. All of its books are created to help families learn how to cope with life's unexpected changes. And, above all, each book is designed to show, in compassionate and intelligent terms, that you, the reader, are not alone.

ACKNOWLEDGMENTS

I would like to thank Richard Scrushy, Pat Foster, Brad Hale and Gerald Nix of HealthSouth for their continued support and help in making HealthSouth Press a success. I would also like to thank Gray Richardson, Tim Robinson, Joyce Roy and the entire art staff of HealthSouth Press for their talent, expertise, and hard work.

Patricia Brown of HealthSouth RIOSA has been invaluable these last 15 years in always keeping things running smoothly.

And a special thanks goes to Karla Dougherty. Without her this book would not have been written.

CONTENTS

FOREWORD

Multiple sclerosis challenges all who are touched by it. This frustrating and frightening, often progressive disease elicits intense emotional responses, while demanding ongoing adaptation to changes in everyday life. Perhaps the most difficult aspect of the disease is the unpredictability it brings to people's lives. Men and women with MS tell us that one of their greatest challenges is dealing with the constant uncertainty and anxiety about future disability.

In *Multiple Sclerosis: A New Journey,* Dr. Senelick has addressed these issues from a very practical perspective. He provides information that communicates an understanding of the problems encountered, as well as specific measures to address and try to overcome these difficulties. The book discusses the experiences of people with MS and their families from the time of diagnosis through the often tumultuous disease course. The author describes the full range of problems, and suggests an impressive array of potential interventions. The information is conveyed with both sensitivity and humor, creating a genuinely warm document that will help people accept the essential but difficult information they need to know.

This book offers comprehensive information about MS and the complex interventions needed to manage it. It is a valuable resource for people with MS and their families.

Nancy J. Holland, Ed.D.
Vice President
Professional Resource Center & Clinical Programs
National Multiple Sclerosis Society

A New Look
At a Well-Worn Road

It seems like the worst has happened. The symptoms you have been having—the tingling in your hands, the numbness on your left side, the vision problems—they aren't just in your head. They are real. They are there. They haven't just gone away, never to return. They've come back . . . again. And they are much more serious than you thought.

Your doctor referred you to a neurologist who examined you and had an MRI scan done to see what was going on in your brain. It was what he expected, but what he wished wasn't so. . . .

You have MS. Multiple sclerosis. That disease that Martin Sheen's presidential character has on The West Wing. *That condition you've heard about, the one that your aunt, or your distant cousin, or a friend of a friend lives with. The disease without a cure. The disease that will not go away. Never. Only get worse . . . and worse.*

Stop!

Developing multiple sclerosis in today's world does not have to be a bleak, grim journey. It does not have to be the start of a road that only spirals down. It does not have to be a mystery that can't be solved.

Today multiple sclerosis can be treated and stabilized, its course altered.

MS: MORE COMMON THAN YOU THINK

When someone has a severe brain or spinal cord injury, it is catastrophic. The world stops for the survivor, the family, and loved ones near and far. Because these are such dramatic events, they get a great deal of attention—from physicians, hospitals, research facilities, and the press.

Multiple sclerosis is different. Its symptoms are subtle; sometimes people aren't even aware of anything more than a slight discomfort or tingling sensation. It is an unpredictable disease, often receding without any residual symptoms—and sometimes not coming back for years. Other times, MS recedes and reoccurs with great frequency.

Because of the subtle mysteries that cloak MS, it does not get the same attention as a catastrophic accident or disease. This might give people the sense that it is a rare condition— and when you do get it, you might feel even more alone or "picked on" than you would with a different disease.

Nothing could be further from the truth. Multiple sclerosis is a fairly common condition, with approximately 350,000 people who have it living in the United States.

Some other truths—and other "multiple" myths exposed:

Multiple Myth #1: Multiple sclerosis is a fatal disease. Once diagnosed, your fate is sealed.
Not true! Most of those 350,000 people who are diagnosed with MS go on to live as long as anybody else and have a nearly normal life span.

Multiple Myth #2: If you've been diagnosed with MS, you will eventually be paralyzed and in a wheelchair. That's a guarantee.

Yes, it is true that half the people who have multiple sclerosis will eventually have trouble walking. But that fate is not etched in stone. Early detection and early treatment can help improve the odds that you will either delay that time or be the other half that walks independently.

Multiple Myth #3: With MS, it's diagnose—and adios. There's nothing anyone—including your doctor—can do to help.

Wrong again. It's true that in the past doctors were at a standstill when it came to multiple sclerosis. By the time they were able to diagnose it, the disease was in place. There was nothing anyone could do but hope it didn't progress too quickly. That's not true today. The new ABC + R drugs (Avonex®, Betaseron®, Copaxone®, and Rebif®) aggressively treat MS nerve inflammation and help prevent the disease from getting worse. And better diagnostic tools, including today's MRI (magnetic resonance imaging) scan of the brain, mean that MS can be detected very early on. Together, they are a formidable enemy that can keep MS at bay! Add a healthy diet and regular exercise and there's no reason why a person with multiple sclerosis can't have a good quality of life.

Multiple Myth #4: MS is contagious.
No way! There is absolutely no evidence that MS can be passed on from person to person, either through sexual or casual contact. It is not an infectious disease.

Multiple Myth #5: Once a woman is diagnosed with MS, she can forget about getting pregnant and having children.
Wrong again. Not only can a woman with MS get pregnant and give birth, she can even enjoy sex! A severe disability may make pregnancy more difficult, but not impossible. Although relapses are more common in the first few months after delivery, most women will not have a relapse during the pregnancy itself. In fact, most people with multiple sclerosis can have a fulfilling sex life—despite a disability. *(We'll be going over sexuality and multiple sclerosis later in this book.)*

These are only a few of the "multiple" myths around. There are as many myths about multiple sclerosis as there are for other diseases and conditions.

As we all know, fear, especially of the unknown, breeds false theories, and a victim mentality. *Multiple Sclerosis: A New Journey* was written to help dissolve that fear with knowledge and education. It explains what MS is and why it creates its sometimes unpredictable symptoms. This book is your guide to these different symptoms—and the problems you might encounter. You'll learn how to cope with MS and:

- Sexuality
- Your daily life and work routines
- Bladder and bowel function
- Mobility

- Fatigue
- Depression
- Problems with memory and other cognitive functions
- Visual problems
- Spasticity
- Pain

A NEW HOPE, A NEW JOURNEY

Consider *Multiple Sclerosis: A New Journey* your guide to a new landscape, one that tells it "like it is"—while, at the same time, providing real hope, real promise, and real treatment plans.

You'll learn all about the new, effective ways to diagnose multiple sclerosis, biomedical advancements that enable neurologists to better determine *right from the start* whether or not you have MS. It also details everything you need to know about the new, exciting treatments for multiple sclerosis. You'll discover the facts about the disease-modifying drugs (called ABC + R), the medicines that make it possible to fight back aggressively. Between the new diagnostic advances and the ABC + R drugs, your condition can be caught early—and aggressively treated.

You'll also find important information about rehabilitation—and why it is important in promoting a good quality of life. You'll learn what makes a good MS rehabilitation center, the "A-team" health care professionals that work best, even about new alternative therapies that people have tried.

You'll also hear true-life stories of people who have MS—and how they have handled the progression of their disease. You'll find people who have had only two episodes; others who have gotten progressively worse; still others who were never bothered by MS again. You'll feel their hope, their strength, and find real solutions to the real problems that you may have.

Finally, the unique *Multiple Sclerosis: A New Journey* wants you to have the most up-to-the-minute information about MS diagnosis, treatment, research, and symptom management. With that in mind, this book will be updated and revised periodically so that the newest facts and figures will never be more than a page away.

A NEW LOOK AT MULTIPLE SCLEROSIS
FOR PATIENTS AND THEIR LOVED ONES

Statistics show that MS is the leading disease-causing disability in young people. They also show that within 15 years, half the people with MS will not be able to walk without an assistive device.

Change these numbers. Learn everything you can. And, if you have symptoms of MS, don't let them rule you.

This book shows you how to become master of your own disease, your own guide on a journey of hope.

Don't be afraid: be armed.

Let's begin. . . .

PART ONE

THE JOURNEY BEGINS

WHAT IS MULTIPLE SCLEROSIS —AND WHY DID IT HAPPEN TO ME?

*No, I never wished for MS. Just like no one would
wish for cancer or any other disease. But I have it.
It's a fact of my life. What can I do? Crumble and feel
sorry for myself? Or try to live well and strong
and with dignity. I choose the latter. I just need
to know how to do it. . . .*

—A 32-year-old mother of three
recently diagnosed with MS

When Jayne left the advertising agency on Michigan Avenue, she wanted to run all the way down the stairs. She wanted to shout and dance and wave her arms with glee. She got it! A job with one of the biggest advertising agencies in Chicago. It was an entry-level position as an assistant to an account executive, but she didn't care. She'd work hard, learn everything she could, and who knew where she might end up. The agency had branches all over the world. Maybe she would head the Paris office. Or set up accounts in Melbourne, Australia. Who knew!

Everyone Jayne called was impressed with her good news. After all, she'd just graduated from the University of Chicago less than two months ago, and even with layoffs, stiff competition, and her lack of experience, she snagged the job.

Jayne's world was definitely looking good right about now, just about perfect—except for one thing. A minor thing, a slight thing, something she didn't even bother mentioning to her roommate or her boyfriend.

It was her eyes. When she read over the letters she'd typed, or notes about a new ad campaign, or even one of the mystery novels she loved so much, she felt this ache in her left eye. Not exactly in her eye, but behind it, as if it were in her head. She also noticed that she had trouble reading with her left eye; the words blurred, and her vision dimmed.

But Jayne had just started her new job. There was so much to learn, so much to do. She chose to ignore the problem. It persisted, however, and finally Jayne called her eye doctor. The first available lunch-hour appointment was not for two weeks.

During those two weeks, Jayne was tempted to cancel her appointment. Although her eyes bothered her a lot in the beginning, she now barely felt any pain. It was probably a sty, or strain, or just nerves.

But Jayne kept the appointment. Her parents had taught her to take good care of her eyes and encouraged regular eye exams. So, two weeks later, feeling slightly ridiculous, Jayne came into her eye doctor's office.

Her ophthalmologist listened to her story; he didn't discount her problems at all. Instead, he gave her a thorough eye examination, peering at the back of her eyes after her pupils had been dilated for maximal viewing. He noticed a slight swelling of the optic nerve; a visual field test showed an enlargement of the blind spot, the area of the retina that is attached to the optic nerve.

The ophthalmologist put down his diagnostic tools and told Jayne what he'd suspected when she'd first told him her story: She had optic neuritis—an inflammation of the optic nerve, a bundle of nerve fibers that transmits images from the retina to the parts of the brain associated with vision.

Jayne was relieved—at least initially. When she had first experienced her eye pain, she was terrified that she had a brain tumor. She didn't have cancer and she knew that her problems weren't "all in her head". She could breathe again and go back to enjoying her life. After all, the problem had all but disappeared, and with some anti-inflammatory medicine, she'd be as good as new!

Wrong. Her ophthalmologist went on to tell Jayne that optic neuritis is a possible sign of multiple sclerosis, that she had a 50% chance of developing MS. He wanted her to see a neurologist.

Jayne was devastated. Her perfect life was falling apart. All she could think about was Mrs. Forester who lived next door to her parents. Mrs. Forester had been in a wheelchair as long as Jayne had known her; she sometimes slurred her speech, and she looked old before her time. And Mrs. Forester had MS! Would that be Jayne's fate as well? Goodbye advertising job. Goodbye getting married and having a baby. Goodbye traveling and seeing the world. . . .

Jayne was being overly dramatic, letting her imagination get the best of her. There was a reason her dad always kidded her about being "an actress in a Greek tragedy". But imaginary or not, to Jayne the fears felt completely real. She could barely concentrate on work while she waited for her appointment to see the neurologist.

Jayne's fears turned out to be unwarranted. The neurologist had an MRI brain scan performed, and there were no other lesions (abnormal spots) present in her brain. She couldn't have *multiple* sclerosis because she did not have *multiple* lesions.

But Jayne was only 21 years old. It was possible that she could develop MS down the road. She would have to learn to live with a certain amount of uncertainty; she would have to make regular appointments with a neurologist.

Jayne still enjoyed every moment of her life, perhaps even more so. But she had also grown up, taking responsibility for herself. She spent some of her leisure time learning about MS; she tried to live a healthy, fit life.

Although uncertainty was in Jayne's cards, she had taken control of her life. Uncertainty was merely another factor, like career goals, next year's vacation, and favorite foods. It didn't loom large. Jayne had fought her fear—and she had won.

Jayne's story is a typical one. Multiple sclerosis usually begins with a single episode—usually involving the eyes or a "tingly, numb" sensation in the hands or feet—in early adulthood. Fifty to 70% of all people who experience optic neuritis go on to develop MS. In some cases, it might be years before an episode reoccurs—or never. On the other hand, it might reoccur only one month later. MS is an unpredictable disease. Its complexities, its refusal to stay on the straight and narrow, can make it difficult to diagnose.

But early diagnosis is crucial to have an impact on the progression of MS. Is this a Catch-22? A no-win situation? No. Today we know specific facts about MS; we *can* catch it early and, even better, treat it aggressively before it gets worse.

Knowledge is key—your doctor's expertise and your own. This chapter will give you a clear picture of MS: what it is and what it is not.

Let's start with what might have been MS long ago—as we take a step back in time. . . .

A HISTORY LESSON

Although multiple sclerosis—and neurological disease in general—were unknown terms until fairly recently, there's evidence that multiple sclerosis may have been with us for centuries.

The ancient civilizations relied on superstition and magic to "cure" people and exorcise the "evil spirit" who, in their minds, caused a young pharaoh to, perhaps, hobble with a cane, or, say, an aristocratic young bride in Pompeii to slowly lose her ability to see the colorful murals painted on her dining room wall. In reality, the evil spirit was most likely an episode of MS.

Even the ancient Egyptians, who observed and carefully analyzed scientific methods, believed it was the heart that was the center of a person's personality; it was the heart, they believed, that gave people the ability to think. The brain, and any possible lesions, was discarded during the mummification process.

Documents from the Middle Ages are more specific. They describe people who have multiple sclerosis: slurred speech, uneven gait, tremors and numbness, loss of sight.

These early descriptions can only come to us in broad strokes. It wasn't until the 19th century, when scientific methods were adopted, written down, and scrutinized, that multiple sclerosis officially made its way into the annals of medical disease.

In 1868 Jean-Martin Charcot, often called the "father of neurology," happened to examine a young woman who had an unusual tremor. Charcot was intrigued because the tremor was combined with slurred speech and abnormal eye movement. He couldn't help the young woman, but when she died, he performed an autopsy and discovered the characteristic plaques, or lesions, in her brain that we now know signal multiple sclerosis.

But Dr. Charcot was not only intrigued with multiple sclerosis—he was also frustrated. He had no idea how a person contracted MS. Nor did he know how to treat it—and he tried everything: electrical stimulation, strychnine, gold and silver injections, all the treatments that were used to help nerve disorders.

But Dr. Charcot was hindered by his times. There was only so much he could do to understand the disease. It would take the 20th century, with its advances in biotechnology and clinical research, to help researchers better understand what multiple sclerosis was—and how it eroded the nervous system.

Almost an entire century passed from the time the first nerve cells were visually enhanced under a microscope to the clinical trials that proved that MS episodes could be relieved with steroids. In between were many relevant discoveries, including the role of myelin, the sheath that "covers" almost every nerve cell; genetic properties that may make a person predisposed to disease; and viral attacks that turned a person's own immune system against itself.

Fast forward to 1984, in England, when the MRI—a machine that could show brain abnormalities better than any x-ray—was perfected. Now multiple sclerosis lesions could be easily identified and pinpointed; they appeared right there on the computer screen in stark black and white. Finally MS could be recognized for what it was through simple diagnostic procedures.

By the 1990s the extremely effective "ABC + R" drugs were approved by the Food and Drug Administration, and a whole new generation of people with MS learned new facts and envisioned new hope.

A long way from the ancient days of hobbled young pharaohs and nearly blind toga-wearing matrons.

SO . . . NOW WHAT?

Now that you've traveled back in time and learned how it emerged as a real disease, it's time to understand exactly what it is. Thanks to all those inroads in science and medicine, we now have some answers.

MS is one of the most common neurological diseases around—and yet its exact cause is not known. Scientists believe it is a combination of a pre-genetic disposition and a trigger from the environment, perhaps a virus that attacks the immune system and turns it against the nerve cells in your body.

Any disease that affects the central nervous system (CNS) is insidious—and multiple sclerosis is no exception. The CNS is made up of the brain and the spinal cord. Together and apart, they govern the way we think, the way we move, the way we speak. The CNS deals with the sublime by creating the images we dream and providing the strategies to make them real. On the other hand, it also dictates our basic, primal, human needs, such as bladder and bowel function, swallowing, and sexuality.

Unlike a brain trauma or a spinal cord injury, nerves are not suddenly severed in MS, creating abrupt disturbances in the way messages are sent to and from our spinal cord and brain. Instead, multiple sclerosis attacks the myelin, or insulation, that surrounds most nerve fibers in our central nervous system. This myelin helps makes messages course through our brain much more efficiently; it makes sure the message, "Ouch, the stove is hot. Take your finger away!" is sent to your thumb much faster. It helps the brain assimilate the message, "What a gorgeous guy. I hope he looks at me," much faster so that you can quickly understand and act: "Smile and wave now—before he turns away!"

When this myelin becomes inflamed or erodes, these messages are sideswiped. The electrical impulses that carry these messages to the brain don't always make it—or they make it much less efficiently. Symptoms, like Jayne's optic neuritis, or tremors, or cognitive difficulties, can crop up.

But multiple sclerosis doesn't happen overnight. It is a progressive disease. The "multiple" refers to multiple episodes—as well as multiple lesions in the brain. If you only have one lesion, like Jayne, you may not have multiple sclerosis. It may take time to know for certain.

Multiple sclerosis also takes a circuitous route. Unlike a tumor, which continues to grow, or a bruise that starts to bloom black and blue, MS may stop, then not reoccur for years. Or it may leave residual symptoms—that get worse with each ensuing episode. On the other hand, serious symptoms might show up right from the start.

Why? We're not sure—but we are learning. According to the National Multiple Sclerosis Society, today we do know that:

- Multiple sclerosis usually first strikes between the ages of 20 and 50. It is rare before the age of 15 and after 60.
- Twice as many women get MS than men.
- MS is rare in African-Americans and other ethnic groups. It is most common in those of northern European ethnicity.

- MS is the leading disease-causing disability in young people today.
- The further north you live from the equator—and the further south—the more likely you are to develop MS.
- If you move from a northern state, say Michigan for example, to a southern state, such as Florida, before the age of 15, your risk is as low as a Florida native . . .
- But if you move from a northern state *after* the age of 15, the risk remains high—wherever you live.
- Within 15 years after symptoms first appear, 50% of the people with MS will need help in walking, either by using a cane, a wheelchair, or a scooter.
- If detected early—right after the first episode—MS can be treated aggressively and often successfully.

Yes, MS is a serious disease. There is no doubt about it. But we can try to do something about it. However, before we can understand and fight a disease, we have to know its roots. We have to know how it affects our bodies—and where. Thus, we first need to see how the brain and spinal cord work in tandem. We need to know what the immune system is and how it works.

Putting these pieces of the puzzle together will help you navigate your own MS journey more effectively. It will help you understand in depth what multiple sclerosis is—and what you can do to stop it in its tracks.

Get ready for anatomy lesson 101. . . .

CHAPTER TWO

THE HOME OF MS: THE CENTRAL NERVOUS SYSTEM

*Multiple sclerosis? I didn't have a clue what it meant.
Hey, I didn't even care much about my brain or any
part of my anatomy—as long as everything was
working! And the immune system? Forget about it.
But that all changed when I was diagnosed with MS.
I now know everything—and learn something new
every day. I'm a walking encyclopedia, a Ph.D. without the degree. And it's a good thing, too. The more I
know, the better I can control my disease.*

—A 42-year-old policeman who has had
multiple sclerosis for five years

Martha was a typical suburban homemaker. She did some
part-time reception work at the neighborhood community
center, but basically her full-time job was taking care of she
and her husband's three young children. If she wasn't carpooling a bunch of kids to a soccer game in her white SUV,
she was taking one of her own kids to piano lessons or gym-
nastics or a math tutor. She once tried to figure out the
mileage in a typical day—and she gave up after she got to
four complete rounds of the huge mall outside of town. And
that didn't even include going grocery shopping, doing the
laundry, cooking dinner, getting to the dry cleaners, or doing
errands for herself!

Normally, Martha did just fine—even with her busy schedule. She loved her kids and she loved her life. She always had

had a lot of energy, ever since she was a child. And now, at 34, it was still there. No matter how exhausting her day, Martha always had time after dinner to help with homework or talk to her husband about his day.

Lately, though, she'd been feeling exhausted. More nights than not, her husband Jeff had been the one to tuck the children in and read them a story. He'd even washed the dinner dishes—which, more times than not, had become fast-food takeout. Martha just didn't have the energy to cook.

Even then, Martha didn't see any reason to be concerned. After all, she had good reason to be tired!

But then the numbness and tingling began in her legs. It was as if her legs had fallen asleep—but that was impossible. She'd been running around like a maniac trying to get her house ready for a dinner party. There was no way she had sat still long enough for her legs to get "pins and needles."

Worse, whenever she picked up the phone, she found herself slurring her speech; her girlfriend on the other end asked if she was drunk!

Martha did fine at the dinner party; she wasn't totally up to par, but no one really noticed. Her balance was slightly off as she carried platters in from the kitchen, her leg still felt tingly, and her voice was occasionally slurred, but no one really noticed. They were having too good a time.

But Martha knew that something wasn't right. She made an appointment to see her doctor the next day.

The doctor agreed: Something wasn't right. With the tingly, numb feeling, the slurred speech, and the difficulty with balance all pointing to a neurological problem, she sent Martha to a neurologist.

During Martha's first appointment with the neurologist, he asked for a detailed history. He asked if she'd ever had these symptoms before. Martha thought about it for a moment, then remembered that time back in college, about 15 years ago, when she felt numb and tingly on the right side of her face; the feeling radiated down the right side of her body and it lasted about two weeks. She'd been scared that she had had a brain tumor or something, but the school physician assured her it was just stress. Finals were about to begin and everyone was nervous; he'd been seeing symptoms of stress—the headaches, the numbness, the fatigue, the mood swings—in everyone all week. Since Martha's symptoms stopped just about the time her finals were finished, she assumed the school physician was right.

And then came graduation, a brief stint teaching elementary school, marriage, and her three children. Who could remember an incident of "nerves" from so many years ago! It had been long forgotten—until now.

The neurologist ordered an MRI for Martha, one that was enhanced with a chemical called gadolinium. This would give him clearer, more diagnostic views of her brain. When he put the films up on the screen, he saw confirmation of what he had suspected: There were multiple bright white spots, or lesions, on both sides of Martha's brain. There was also a long lesion in her spinal cord near where her shoulder met her neck (called the thoracic area).

The evidence was clear: Martha definitely had multiple sclerosis. She had had *multiple* (at least two) episodes within her lifetime and she had *multiple* lesions in her central nervous system.

Martha and Jeff made an appointment to meet with their neurologist two days after the confirmed diagnosis. They needed to discuss Martha's options. But before the visit, they bombarded the Internet. They wanted to know as much as they could about this disease. They wanted to be able to make an informed decision when they meet with the doctor.

Fortunately for Martha and Jeff, the neurologist was able to answer every single one of their questions. He was even more up-to-date with the information on the Internet than they were. As the director of a comprehensive multiple sclerosis center, their neurologist was better informed than many other doctors in private practice. In addition to giving them several brochures and booklets, he discussed the full complement of literature to help them understand their options.

Finally, a decision was made: Martha would begin a five-day course of high-dose steroids infused via injection into her veins—which would shorten the length of her current episode. To keep her symptoms at bay, Martha would continue taking a smaller dose of steroids by mouth for the next ten days.

The course of action worked. Martha came back for her follow-up visit two weeks later, feeling better and healthy. One of the booklets her doctor had given her explained all about the new ABC+R drugs, a group of disease-modifying drugs that had recently been proved to help prevent future relapses of her multiple sclerosis. Both Martha and her neurologist agreed that she'd be a good candidate to give one of them a try.

Today, five years later, Martha's kids have left soccer afternoons for SAT tutors. Martha still keeps up her hectic schedule, but she remembers to add in nap times and to delegate some of the carpooling and meal planning. She takes her disease-modifying drug regularly and doesn't miss a dose. Jeff does more of the household chores and even the kids have joined in. She does aqua aerobics at her local YMCA pool and she makes sure she eats plenty of fruits and vegetables. She has joined a local chapter of the National Multiple Sclerosis Society and attends a support group once a month.

Martha has been healthy and has not had a recurring episode of MS since the time it was diagnosed. That doesn't mean she won't have another episode ever—but, if she does, she is prepared. She has the best possible medical care, she has the knowledge she needs to make informed decisions, and she has a loving, supportive family. Martha feels very fortunate!

Martha's story is not unusual. From the way she first discovers she has multiple sclerosis to its hopeful ending, this story is a common one. Many people don't get diagnosed with the disease until they've had a second episode—some time after the first one had been dismissed as nerves, or stress, or "all in the head."

But wouldn't it be wonderful if the story could start out different—if the first episode could be diagnosed as MS with an MRI and if the appropriate drugs could be given right from the start.

This can happen only with education. And that's what this chapter—indeed, this whole book—is about: learning. We will take you inside your head and your spinal column. We will give you a basic anatomy lesson so you can know the main "players" involved in MS and understand their rules.

IF I ONLY HAD A BRAIN . . .

By itself, the brain doesn't look like much: a wet, moldy brown sponge. In fact, the ancient Egyptians thought it was so useless that they pulled it out of the head during the embalming process.

But don't let appearances fool you. The brain is more complex, more organized and efficient, more able to store and retrieve information than the most micro-chipped, most cutting-edge computer Bill Gates could ever imagine. That supposedly "useless sponge" contains millions and millions of neurons, or nerve cells, connected to each other by an electrochemical highway that takes messages to and from every single part of our body—from our eyes and our nose to our little fingers and our toes.

This highway is a busy one: Think rush hour at Christmas time. And there are many "stops" or locales along this brain highway—and within the entire nervous system as well—where messages might pause for a moment, rest and observe, stay for the night, or settle in for life.

Let's take a trip on the nerve superhighway—from the very edge of the nervous system to the central port:

STOP 1: THE PERIPHERAL NERVOUS SYSTEM: THE OUTER BANKS

Think of the circuitry behind the outlet by your desk, the "fiber optics" cacophony that the phone companies are always hawking. This maze of wires and cords is very similar to the way your peripheral nervous system looks. It is an intricate, swirling, curling, crowding superhighway of nerves—from the nerve endings in your fingertips to the nerves in your muscles, from the nerves entwined in your organs to the nerves attached to your muscles and your face. These nerves all play a role in transmitting messages to your spinal cord and brain. The hot stove you touch, the ice-cold drink you taste, the nail under your bare foot—all these sensations, or stimuli, travel toward the brain to elicit a response. The brain then sends a message back, and you quickly withdraw the sore foot or the burned finger. But, without the brain's interpretation, the pain or the thirst-quenching feeling would be meaningless; you wouldn't feel or think or remember anything of these or other sensations at all. Think of the peripheral nervous system as an extremely efficient messenger service—one that travels along the superhighway to drop off and deliver a specific message "package": act, feel, think.

STOP 2: THE SPINAL CORD: THE FIRST "MUST SEE" IN THE CENTRAL NERVOUS SYSTEM

The central nervous system. Remember these words. Multiple sclerosis affects the central nervous system (CNS). It is the place where the disease calls home. Damage to the nerve fibers in either the brain or the spinal cord may produce MS symptoms.

The first "stop" in the CNS is the spinal cord, a kind of relay station between your peripheral nervous system and your brain. Messages from the nerves in your fingers that touched a hot stove go up the spinal cord to be interpreted by the brain. The "ouch" of pain, as well as the action response—"Move your fingers pronto!"—travels from the brain back down the spinal cord to those burned fingers. Like the only bridge linking a city with the suburbs, all responses from the brain must go via the spinal cord: to walk, to run, to gesture, to feel, to get out of there now!

There are three crucial spinal "taps", or facts, you need to know to understand some of the symptoms you may experience with MS:

Spinal Tap #1: You Say Vertebrae, I Say Vertebra: The Spinal Column

The brain has its skull for protection. Similarly, the spinal cord also has its "shield": the spinal column, a skeletal frame made up of bony blocks, one on top of the other. These blocks are called vertebrae. (And, just in case you become a contestant on the next big television quiz show, a single block is called a vertebra.)

Intervertebral discs, made of gelatinous material, separate each vertebra block. Along with helping to protect the spinal cord and keep the spinal column flexible, they also help absorb shock by acting as a cushion between each vertebra. These are those selfsame "slipped discs" that can cause excruciating back pain.

The spinal cord—always 18 inches long—runs through and down the stacked vertebrae and intervertebral discs. Medical science has given each vertebra an identifying letter and number—which means that physicians only have to call out the i.d. to immediately pinpoint the exact location of the damage is and what it will be:

√ The "Top Seven" vertebrae are called the cervical vertebrae; they start at the base of the skull and are noted
   as C1 to C7.

√ The next group is the "Twelve Thoracics." These follow
   down from the bottom of the neck through the chest to
   the curve of the back. These are noted, from highest to
   lowest, as T1 to T12.

√ The lower back contains the "Last Lumbars." There are
   five of them: L1 to L5.

√ The spinal column ends at L2, but the spinal cord nerves
   go on. These remaining nerves, dubbed the *cauda
   equina* (which is Latin for "horse's tail," hang down from

L2 to what is called the five Sacrals. These final five vertebrae help protect the "horse's tail" and are fused
together into a tailbone. They are labeled S1 to S5.

√ Last but not least is the coccyx. You'll feel it when
you've sat too long.

Spinal Tap #2: Nerves of Steel: Bundles of Nerves Within and Without the Spinal Column

The spinal cord, nestled in its spinal column, is much more
than a way station for the brain. Brain-bound bundles of
spinal nerves stem from the brain to the lower back; they

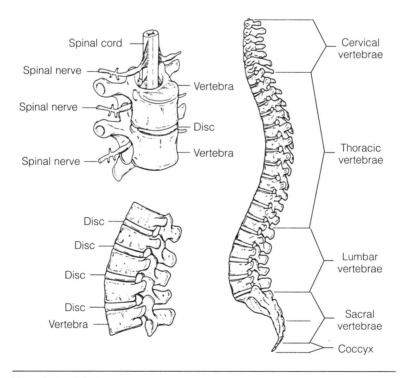

Your Spinal Column

move muscles, joints, and limbs with the help of "orders from above": the brain. There are also spinal nerve fibers in between the bundles of spinal nerve cord that branch out into the peripheral nervous system. These move muscles, joints, and limbs; they are involved in the muscular reflex reactions that require no thought, no brain power, such as the famous "knee jerk reaction"—which was first coined when a doctor lightly tapped a knee—or the equally famous "no-brainer" cliché.

Spinal Tap# 3: A Straight Line From A to B: Location is All

The spinal cord also has functions that can be affected by multiple sclerosis lesions. But unlike the brain, which is very complex, convoluted, and sometimes unpredictable, the spinal cord is very straightforward. "A" always equals "B" when it comes to interpretation.

When the spinal cord is damaged, messages cannot get to the brain. Depending on the location of the nerve damage, specific functions will be affected: the brain just isn't getting it. Messages can't be relayed to the brain and, consequently, the brain can't offer any action, plan, or thought.

Multiple sclerosis lesion damage in the spinal cord can result in muscular problems, weakness, loss of balance and coordination, inability to walk without help. Likewise, the fibers that carry sensations may be affected leading to numbness or loss of sensation below the level of the lesion.

An MS lesion in the neck, for example, may cause problems in the arms and legs, while damage to spinal cord location L1, for example, will result in problems with hip and knee muscles. Damage to the S2 nerve bundles, on the other hand, will result in problems with bladder and bowel.

STOP 3: THE BRAIN: THE BIGGEST TOURIST ATTRACTION ON THE CENTRAL NERVOUS SYSTEM HIGHWAY

Let's add color and dimension to our burned finger and the hot stove. Let's say there's a summer breeze coming through the kitchen window; the sun is fading, a peaceful dusk settles in the backyard; the smell of homemade apple pie is wafting through the rest of the house. These sights and sounds bring you back to a time of innocence and childhood, a time when everyone you loved was safe and sound.

"Ouch!" The finger on the hot stove got its message across, up through the peripheral nervous system and the spinal cord to the brain. The brain is busy; it's not only picking up the finger-stove maneuver, it's also picking up other stimuli from other sensations: the warm breeze, the smell of apple pie, the color of the sky.

These sensation messages, just like the pain of the burned finger, don't just fly directly up to the brain. Although stimulus and reaction messages really do seem to travel up and down faster than the speed of light, the road they take is not a straight one. They pass through various "portals," or sections, of the brain before hitting the "main brain." Let's go over these "portals" now:

Brain Portal #1: The Brainstem

Attached to the spinal cord by thick nerve fibers, the brainstem is home to our most primal basic needs. It is divided into three arenas, the:

- *Medulla,* which is as basic as you can get. Here are the life-sustaining controls for breathing in and breathing out, heart rate, and blood pressure.

- *Pons.* Think of this as a bridge linking the medulla to the higher, more evolved "portals" of the brain. The "tourist attraction" here is the *recticular formation,* a conglomeration of nerve fibers that control muscle tone, reflexes, wakefulness, and the mechanisms that keep you alert and ready to react to change.
- *Midbrain.* You'll find more *recticular formation* action here as well—from staying alert to keeping your reflexes honed. This portion of the brainstem, with the pons, also controls your eye muscles. It's the one portion of the brain we share with all lower animals. (For many animals, this is the final stop on the brain evolution highway.)

Traveling through these three arenas of the brainstem are *all the fibers* that control movement and sensation. A problem here can cause weakness or loss of feeling in the face, arms or legs.

Brain Portal #2: The Cerebellum
Travel behind the brainstem and you'll discover the cerebellum, which regulates all your movements—your balance, your gait, your ability to keep your hand from shaking when you drink a cool soda. Think of the cerebellum as "traffic control." It never fails to keep your movements smooth and coordinated; it even helps smooth and coordinate your speech muscles.

Brain Portal #3: The Cerebrum
This IS the brain, the chunky gray and white matter that makes up what we call the brain.

The gray portion maintains our neurons (nerve cells). It is the area where messages are transported to and from the brain. It is also responsible for the way we think, the way we move, the way we view the world. The gray portion also controls our automatic, instinctual muscle movements that take place in our tongue when we speak, in our eyes when we blink, in our mouth and throat when we chew some of that warm apple pie.

The white matter is more like insulation; it enables the nerve fibers (axons) to send and receive their messages more efficiently and correctly.

Multiple sclerosis doesn't attack the gray matter. *MS is a disease of the white matter in the brain and spinal cord.* It attacks the insulation (myelin)—and the actual message-transmitting apparatus (axons). In attacking these, the very mechanisms that ensures proper "reception," MS can affect your thoughts, your sensations, your memory, your gait, and your balance. The function that is affected depends on where the lesions, or plaques, crop up in the white matter of your brain and spinal cord.

Brain Portal #4: The Hemispheres of the Brain

This is it: the destination at the end of the highway, the place, literally, of your dreams. This is the area of higher-functioning thought, memory, and perception. It is the largest area of the brain—and the one that makes us uniquely human. The *cortex* is the grey lining, that grey-brown color we conjure up when we think of a brain. It is a stretchy, wrinkled blanket made of billions and billions of nerve cells that covers, protects, and clings to the cerebrum—the core of our brain.

Not only are there different areas of the brain, each with its own function, its own "tourist attraction," but there are also two separate halves of the "brain highway." Look in the mirror. Imagine a line going straight down the middle of your head, dividing it into two perfectly equal halves. These two halves, mirror images of each other, are called the left hemisphere and the right hemisphere of the brain. They are connected by the *corpus callosum*, a highway "bridge" rich in nerve cells and fibers. Although both hemispheres are involved in our actions, thoughts, and feelings—with messages being sent to and fro across the *corpus callosum*—each hemisphere does have a "specialty" function that can be

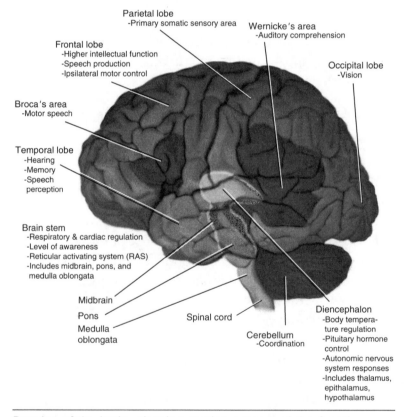

Parietal lobe
-Primary somatic sensory area

Wernicke's area
-Auditory comprehension

Frontal lobe
-Higher intellectual function
-Speech production
-Ipsilateral motor control

Occipital lobe
-Vision

Broca's area
-Motor speech

Temporal lobe
-Hearing
-Memory
-Speech
 perception

Brain stem
-Respiratory & cardiac regulation
-Level of awareness
-Reticular activating system (RAS)
-Includes midbrain, pons, and
 medulla oblongata

Midbrain
Pons
Medulla
oblongata

Spinal cord

Cerebellum
-Coordination

Diencephalon
-Body temperature regulation
-Pituitary hormone control
-Autonomic nervous system responses
-Includes thalamus, epithalamus, hypothalamus

Drawing of the brain, showing section areas and the function they mastermind affected if MS lesions crop up. (Remember, MS affects the "fibers" that connect sections; the nerve cells are fine—they just can't get the message out.)

- *The left hemisphere* is most responsible for language, for speech and word usage. It is the part of the brain most involved in reading, calculating, writing, and other forms of communication. It is also responsible for movement and sensation on the *right* side of the body.
- *The right hemisphere* is the colorful half. It gives language its dash and inflection. It controls your visual memories, your artistic abilities to draw, dance, write, or play music. It is also responsible for your ability to see the bigger, long-term picture. And, like the left is to the right, it is responsible for movement and sensation on the *left* side of the body. (Think of the reflection in a mirror—and how the arm or leg or eye that seems to move is the opposite of the one that's actually moving. It's the same with the brain hemispheres. They truly are mirror images of one another!)

Both sides of the hemisphere are needed to complete a whole. You need the left side of the brain to tell the story of how you burned your finger, the chronology of events, and the way you felt. But the right side of the brain will make it interesting—adding color and description of the room, your grandmother, and your enthusiasm for apple pie.

When an MS lesion appears in one hemisphere, the opposite side of the body will be affected. In other words, if the right hemisphere of your brain has the damage, your left side may be weakened or paralyzed—and vice versa.

Further, emotional symptoms may show up differently, depending where the lesion occurs.

FLOATING ISLAND

The brain does not stand alone. In fact, it floats—in what we call cerebrospinal fluid. This clear water-like liquid surrounds the brain, nourishing it and protecting in much the same way as an airbag protects a passenger in a car. Cerebrospinal fluid also fills the open spaces (called ventricles and cisterns) of the brain. New fluid replaces the old six times a day and within the fluid are chemicals that can be tested to help make an MS diagnosis.

Brain Portal #5: The Lobes of the Brain

Just when you think you've got it down pat, there's more. The brain not only has two complete mirror images of itself, it also is divided into lobes which help define the lobe's function. There are four lobes in each hemisphere, each with different functions, each affecting you in different ways if you develop MS.

- *The frontal lobes* are, of course, in front. They are the lobes of our "higher selves" and they control so much of who we are: impulses, motivation, social interaction, communication, even our voluntary movement. They also give us the ability to retrieve memory from storage as well as house the "brain chip" that is responsible for all movement on the opposite side of the body. In addition, the frontal lobes are home to our "executive functions"—which include our abilities to organize, plan, stay focused, make decisions, and set goals. Damage here can possibly affect a person's cognitive abilities—

hindering attention span, communication, and organizational skills. It can also play havoc with emotions, making a person moody, depressed, or simply "flat".

- *The temporal lobes* nestle above our ears just behind and below the frontal lobes. Here is where the bulk of our memory is stored. They hold our remembrances of both the recent and distant pasts; they hold our learned fund of knowledge and information. Here, too, is the home of the hippocampus and its bounty of emotional thoughts. The temporal lobes give us the ability to understand language and appreciate music. They are also the "processing house" for our perceptions, deciphering what we hear, making sense of incoming information, and sequencing it. Lesions here can affect a person's memory.

- *The parietal lobes* are very "sensitive". Situated just above our ears in the back half of the brain, they are responsible for our sense of touch. They also play a major role in academic abilities; they help us understand what we read and the relationships of where things are in space. Lesions in the parietal lobes can hinder the ability to physically feel and recognize an object. They can also lead to distorted or unusual sensations such as super-sensitivity to touch.

- *The occipital lobe*s control our vision. They are literally "the eyes in the back of our heads." Visual messages start at the back of our eyes on the retina and travel along the optic nerves to the back of the brain. The occipital lobes are the areas where we understand and interpret what we have seen. Inflammation of the optic nerve, optic neuritis, leads to dimming or loss of vision in one eye.

COMMUTING WITHIN THE BRAIN: NEURONS, AXONS, AND MYELIN

We started this journey at the peripheral nervous system. We traveled through the spinal cord and entered the brain. We've learned the different functions of the spinal cord and the different areas of the brain—and which functions are affected if MS attacks a particular part.

At the same time that we've expanded our knowledge of the central nervous system (CNS), we also narrowed our focus, our journey, to the white matter of the brain—specifically the myelin insulation around each nerve cell. This is where MS hits and it is what we will explore next.

DISSECTING A NEURON

Communication is an art, or so some pundits say. But strip away the cocktail party chatter, the surrounding smells and sounds, the other people and their clothes, and you are left with a message that is sent from one person to another—and given a response.

It is no different in the brain. Communication of any message, stripped to its basics, is getting it across, getting it to the right place, and getting an appropriate response.

In the brain and spinal cord, this is done in an amazing thread made up of electrical impulses and hormonal chemicals called neurotransmitters. Messages are relayed throughout the brain and spinal cord by a network of nerve cells, called neurons, the "cables" that conduct messages within them, called axons, and chemical "bridges," the neurotransmitters, that connect one to the other.

Let's go back to that hot stove. Once we've touched the burner, an electrical impulse carrying the "Ouch!" of pain travels through a *nerve receptor* from its outlying *dendrite tentacles* to *a nerve cell body* and out again along the thin "cable" called the *axon*. But as "ouch!" gets to the end of the axon, it runs into a gap called a *synapse*. The next neuron lies in wait, but the electrical charge can't cross the synapse. "Ouch!" would become history at this point if it weren't for an electro-chemical miracle: the electrical impulse that had brought it this far triggers the release of a chemical called the *neurotransmitter* which jumps across the synapse to a *receptor* on the next neuron cell. This starts the electrical conduction down the new axon. "Ouch!" continues on its way until it reaches a new synapse.

In other words:

1. A message in the form of an electrical impulse travels through the dendrite, cell body, and axon of a neuron.
2. The electrical impulse stops at a synapse, or space, between neurons.
3. The electrical impulse triggers the release of the chemical neurotransmitter . . .
4. . . . which "carries" the message across the space to receptors in the new neuron.
5. The electrical impulse continues on its way, through the dendrite, cell body, and axon of the new neuron.
6. The entire process is repeated over and over again until it reaches the part of the brain where the message is intended: neuron to synapse to neuron.
7. A message response repeats the process, neuron to synapse to neuron, as it leaves the various parts of the brain and goes back to the finger: "Get that finger off the stove!"

Now picture this simple-sounding activity occurring all over your CNS at a fast and furious pace, relaying message after countless message to its different areas, deciphering, storing, and shouting commands all at the same time. No pun intended, but it does boggle the mind to think how accurate, how attuned, how precise the human CNS remains, day after day, minute after minute, second after second!

Even more fascinating is the fact that chemical neurotransmitters know which particular electrical charge will give them a "spark" and trigger their release. Like a game of bingo, each neurotransmitter can be triggered by only one "winner", one particular electrical impulse match, in order for the message to jump the synapses. Without the correct electrical impulse message, a chemical neurotransmitter will not be triggered. It will lie dormant, silent, quiet, waiting for its match.

This is all well and good when the brain is functioning normally, when specific messages are being relayed efficiently and correctly. Unfortunately, this efficiency can deteriorate when MS attacks the CNS.

The place it first aims for is the myelin: the protective sheath that covers the majority of axons in the brain and spinal cord.

MYELIN MADNESS

Think of the electrical cords that connect your toaster, your computer, your television, sometimes it seems your very life! None of those cords is bare. Every single one of them is protected by a covering of rubber, plastic, or some other synthetic material. This insulation not only prevents you from getting an electrical shock, it also ensures that the cord, usually a bundle of twisted wires, will work well for a long time.

39

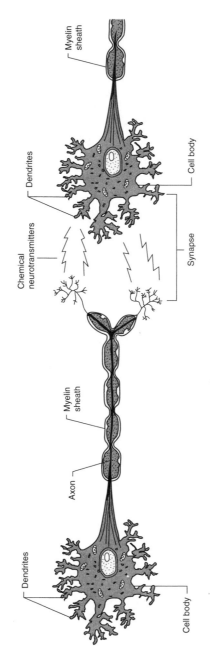

Drawing of an axon covered by the white matter myelin sheath that is primarily affected in Multiple Sclerosis. Neurons connect to axons that carry the message to a synapse and then to other neurons.

This insulation is exactly what myelin is—only the "electrical cords" are within your brain and spinal cord. Myelin in the CNS is made by cells called oligodendrocytes; it is "spun" tightly over the axons, a membrane of insulation, and keeps them running efficiently and healthfully.

But things don't always work out the way they are supposed to. The same goes with our body. Sometimes the very immune system that is designed to protect our body and keep viruses and germs away does the opposite. Sometimes the immune system attacks itself. *(Read more about the immune system and its role in MS in the next chapter.)*

This is exactly what happens in multiple sclerosis. The immune system attacks and destroys first the oligodendrocytes, the cells that make myelin. It goes on to attack the myelin sheath, and, ultimately, the disease attacks the axon and the nerve cell itself.

As soon as the myelin sheaths are attacked, they become inflamed. The result? Electrical impulses that cannot be efficiently transferred from neuron to neuron. Messages become "lost" or misinterpreted. Function at the lesion site becomes confused and disabled.

And the more severe the inflammation, the more intense the symptoms of multiple sclerosis will likely be.

But there is hope. Research is actually pinpointing possible treatment to the oligodendrocyte cells themselves, impacting the progression of MS in its early stages.

And, in the meantime, there are powerful drugs: the ABC + Rs that may delay damage to the myelin sheaths and axons, and keep multiple sclerosis at bay.

But before we go into the treatment of MS, we still have a villain to recognize: an autoimmune system that attacks itself.

CHAPTER THREE

WHEN GOOD BECOMES EVIL: THE ROLE OF THE IMMUNE SYSTEM IN MS

I felt awful, as if there was something about me that was defective. I was hurting myself and couldn't do anything about it. Who would think that the immune system, which is supposed to take care of us, turns on us instead? It's like a switch going off in the night—in the wrong room. Thanks to my doctors, I know it's not my fault, something I did or didn't do. I just have to take care of it, that's all. And I am.

—A 38-year-old female accountant with MS
who is on disease-modifying drug therapy

When Molly was diagnosed with multiple sclerosis, the first thing she did was check out the Internet. She found dozens of sites for multiple sclerosis, with information on everything from the different categories of MS to the different treatments. She found support groups, chat rooms, alternative medicine theories, clinical studies, pharmaceutical treatments, rehabilitation techniques, and quality-of-life issues.

Molly also learned exactly what multiple sclerosis was: its risk factors and its early symptoms.

Her doctor was helpful as well. A neurologist who specialized in multiple sclerosis, he actively kept up with the newest research and treatment plans. He answered all her questions about the medication she was taking—thoroughly and in-depth. He discussed her symptoms and he explained her MRI scan; he told her the parts of the brain and spinal cord that were affected and what that meant in terms of function.

Molly was a trouper. A single woman who lived alone, she was used to being independent. She worked with her doctor and, armed with information, adapted her life to her new condition.

But one thing bothered Molly. Although she now knew that MS was an autoimmune system disease and that her immune system had turned against itself, she didn't truly understand what that meant. If she were honest with herself, she would say that she didn't really understand what the immune system was—or how it worked. Her doctor tried to explain it to her, but his time was short. He suggested some articles and books, but even those were confusing.

Molly wanted answers. She also wanted to learn. She wanted to discover everything she could about this character who played such a crucial role in her disease.

You, too, might want answers about your own immune system—and how it can attack itself. . . .

IMMUNITY FOR ALL

Our immune system literally saves our lives, tirelessly seeking out alien viruses, bacteria, and germs that have invaded our bodies. It is our body's first line of defense.

Its name, like so many other medical terms, comes from the Latin: "auto" means oneself, and "immune" means exactly that: your immune system, the vast network of antibodies and white blood cells that fight off those virulent invaders.

Your immune system has two main components: your blood, specifically your white blood cells, and the cells that comprise your body.

Let's go inward, a "side-trip" so to speak, and journey inside our bodies, becoming smaller and smaller, until we've entered a cell. Since this a book about MS, let's make it an oligodendrocyte, the cell that makes myelin. *(In actuality, it can be any cell; this chapter explains how the immune system works in general to keep your body healthy.)*

ENTER YOUR CELL AND ITS THE PROTECTIVE SHIELD

The protective cell membrane that covers each cell (including an oligodendrocyte), is a feat of engineering to rival the gadgetry in the newest Syms® computer game. It's a semipermeable shell with no hinges, no doors, and no locks; it only allows certain substances in—and keeps undesirable materials out.

It's all done by code—which is determined by the patterns of our genetic structure. In addition to spelling out the color of our eyes, our height, and our predilection for hot stoves and warm apple pie, these gene patterns create and inhabit every cell of our body. They also happen to stud the outer surface of every cell, in our case, oligodendrocytes. Similar gene patterns are recognized as friends; they can enter and leave the cell at will; they are welcome guests. But viruses—which are nothing more than floating scraps of DNA, genetic garbage that hasn't been thrown out—have unusual, strange patterns. In an ideal world, the wall of the oligodendrocyte would be shut tight to these virus scraps, and they'd never get past the outer membrane.

But cells, even our hearty oligodendrocytes, are not always vigilant. Viruses can sometimes "slip" through a cell's wall. Perhaps the DNA protein that covers a virus is not recognized as an enemy. Perhaps there are so many virus scraps floating around that one or two will get through unnoticed. Or perhaps the immune system is busy working overtime on something else, an open cut or a congested chest, and it doesn't notice the virus entering the oligodendrocyte.

However the virus enters, there is still good news. A virus that enters a cell can still be discovered and destroyed—thanks to the killer instinct of our immune system.

ENTER YOUR IMMUNE SYSTEM
AND VISIT ITS VIGILANT SOLDIERS

When a virus comes into a cell, any cell, including an oligo-dendrocyte, it leaves a "jacket" on the cell's surface. This jacket is a pattern of DNA protein that signals an illegal entry to our immune system army. This molecular "jacket" is called an *antigen.*

While this antigen is getting comfortable and settling in, the immune system soldiers—all two million or so killer cells called *lymphocytes* that are encamped in your lymph nodes—are getting ready for the hunt.

Each lymphocyte seeks out alien cell surfaces as it travels through your body. As a lymphocyte races through your bloodstream, it "touches" the cells it passes; it can feel an antigen's "jacket." But it is selective. Like a key in a lock, a piece in a puzzle, only one specific lymphocyte will hone in and connect to only one specific antigen.

There are three types of lymphocytes in the immune system arsenal:

Surface-to-Air Missiles: B-Cells
These lymphocytes are created in our bone marrow and they specialize in detecting antigens at a distance. They not only

recognize by "touch", but they also send out "missile" anti-bodies that travel through the bloodstream to seek out aliens. They can fight and kill bacteria and viruses before they've had a chance to get close to a cell. B-cells are by far the most numerous of all lymphocytes.

The Secret Weapon: Immunoglobulin (Ig)

The official name for the antibody "missile" sent out by the B-cells is immunoglobulin (Ig). Faster and faster, one after another, at a rate of about 2,000 per minute, the Igs are unleashed into the bloodstream. They put their mark on alien-invaded cells as they zoom by. These marks are powerful chemical enzymes that coat infected cells, creating a rich "syrup." Nearby phagocytes, the scientific name for white blood cells, are attracted by the scent. Like bees to honey, they gobble up these alien-invaded cells—irrevocably destroying them in a flash of chemical reaction. One for the Igs!

Ground Control: T-Cells

T-cells are not as common a lymphocyte as B-cells and their Ig sidekicks, but they are no less deadly. T-cells do their detecting at close quarters, honing in on cells that have already been invaded. They originate in the thymus gland—which sits just underneath our breastbone.

MEMORY: YOUR IMMUNE SYSTEM'S "SECRET WEAPON" TO WARD OFF DISEASE

Here's a sobering fact: When a person gets infected with a virus, the vast majority of his immune cells are, at first, help-less to detect and destroy it. Only a few "wise" lymphocytes can recognize the virus and make a feeble attempt to kill it.

But experience is everything. Once the virus is no longer a stranger, the immune cells, as they continuously divide and replicate from their original mother cell, begin to recognize it. They remember.

Now that the immune cells know their enemy, they can fight. The lymphocytes zero in on the alien-invaded cells and "glom" onto them. They stop them in their tracks before they can do any more damage. The result? You might not succumb to that pneumonia again—or, in other words, been there, done that. You might just end up with just a common cold.

This is what our immune system is all about: the body healing itself. Unfortunately, even with this terrific weaponry, a virus can get the better of our immune system. Once a virus has entered a cell, it can "hide" from the body army—even with its antigen "jacket" waving in the membrane breeze. The virus scrap can live inside a cell without the surrounding cells being the wiser. It can grow and grow and create thousands of virus clones before it is detected and T-cells, B-cells, and the Igs are called up.

But, by this time, the thousands of replicated virus clones could have easily slipped into the surrounding cells—and given birth to an illness—from colitis to Plantar's warts, from meningitis to, in a worst case scenario, various forms of cancer.

THE SELF-SABOTAGE PHENOMENON: YOUR AUTOIMMUNE SYSTEM AND MS

So now you've met your autoimmune system: a strong army that is always on alert. The perfect soldiers who, if they happen not to recognize an enemy initially, will never let it happen again. Perfect, strong, efficient. A fast, smooth vehicle that makes your journey a healthy one.

But sometimes things happen. In an ironic twist of fate, your immune system can turn on itself. Your body literally begins to battle its own cells—mistaking your healthy, robust cells as the enemy. This is exactly what happens in MS: Your B-cells, T-cells, and Igs start attacking the oligodendrocyte cells that make myelin. Eventually the immune system attacks not only these cells, but the myelin sheaths themselves. Once these sheaths weaken, the immune system goes to work on the axons in your brain and spinal cord—the very fibers that carry the messages for motor function, mood, perception, and all your activities of daily living. Here's how this self-destructive phenomenon works:

1. The lymphocytes, in their scouting expedition, sound the alarm: an enemy virus has entered our cells!
2. The lymphocytes begin their "touch and search", feeling out each "jacket" on every cell to "flush out" the stranger.
3. B-cells send out their antibody missiles: They head for the oligodendrocyte cells.
4. T-cells also get up close and personal with these cells.
5. For some reason, the oligodendrocyte cells don't seem familiar; the lymphocytes don't recognize them as their own.
6. The lymphocytes go after the oligodendrocyte cells as if they were the enemy: they are on the attack.
7. Your entire autoimmune system is now at war—with itself. It attacks your oligodendrocytes, your myelin sheaths, and the axons of your nerve cells.
8. The result? Multiple sclerosis lesions.

WHY?

Why MS? Why do some people get it and not others? The answers are not all in, but we do believe that it is not the result of a particular virus that enters the body. Rather, it is a *combination* of an environmental "trigger" (a virus that enters the body and/or the geographical location of an individual) and certain genetic predispositions, such as gender and family history. *(See chapter one for the risk factors for MS).*

ALL IN THE FAMILY

The family connection may be a clue to why some people get MS. Studies have found that if one identical twin develops multiple sclerosis, the other twin has a 31% chance of getting it as well. For siblings who are not twins, the chances are lower: only three to five percent. Although that number might be small, it's important to remember that the risk is still 20 to 40 times higher than the normal population.

Knowing where MS takes root is not enough. Understanding your risks—as well as brain, spinal cord, and immune system—is only half the story. You need to know how to detect MS—and how it journeys through your body. We've tried to explain the "Why" in this section. Next, we'll tackle the "How."

PART TWO

THE HIGHWAY SIGNS

CHAPTER FOUR

READING THE SIGNS: EARLY SYMPTOMS OF MS

I knew something was wrong, but I couldn't put my finger on it. My waist sometimes felt weird, like there was a cold fish wrapped around it! It was like I had no sensation there. I'd take a shower and towel off, but I couldn't feel it. I also couldn't open jars the way I used to, even plastic ketchup bottles were tough. I thought it was stress, especially because I was so tired all the time. My wife made me go to the doctor, though—and I'm glad she did. Turns out I had MS.

—A 42-year-old male high school teacher with relapsing-remitting multiple sclerosis

Emily was one of those people who hated to go to doctors. She wasn't afraid to take aspirin, of course, when she had a headache, and she also took a whole slew of vitamins. She ate healthfully: five servings of fruits and vegetables a day, lots of fiber and complex carbohydrates, and very little fat. Emily also drank skim milk and took a calcium supplement every day. She was 38, and she figured you can't start early enough on the road to good health. She wanted a vigorous, energetic old age.

So when she started to feel dizzy, in the middle of the day at her desk, or even walking home from the bus station, Emily tried to ignore it. She simply went about her business.

But the dizziness continued; she felt off-balanced, as if she were sailing on a ship. Worse, she got tired, so tired, that she dreamed of taking a nap in the afternoon. It took all her energy just to sit at her desk; she pretended to be working on a report.

Emily figured it was the dizziness and loss of balance that were making her tired. She stocked up on iron pills, took some ginger for her dizziness, and continued to keep to her schedule as much as she could. She told herself it was nothing.

"I don't need a doctor," she told a friend over lunch. "What's he going to say? You need to rest—and take aspirin. It's probably an allergy or something. I'll be fine." She stabbed at her Cobb salad with such fury that her friend didn't say a word.

And, lo and behold, the symptoms went away. Emily was so relieved. Now, more than ever, she knew she didn't need doctors. She had taken care of the problem herself!

Emily almost seemed to have more energy than she'd had before. She plunged into her routine with a vengeance: an hour at the Y working out, getting to her publishing job by 8:30, working until 7:00, then meeting friends for a drink and dinner. She was exuberant, happy. Emily laughed more than ever.

Two months later, Emily was fastening a skirt when she had the oddest sensation. It was like something cold had wrapped itself around her waist. It wasn't that she couldn't feel her waist; it just felt oddly cool and full. The area felt itchy, but if she tried to scratch herself, the itchiness would not go away.

Emily shrugged and, as she was putting on her shoe, she lost her balance. She had to hold on to the dresser to stop herself from falling to the carpet.

The dizziness had come back in full force—along with the fatigue.

Something was definitely wrong.

But what got Emily to her doctor (the only one she had was a gynecologist) was the bladder problem she developed. She'd occasionally wet herself before making it to the bathroom. She was so embarrassed and upset that she had to call for help.

Emily's gynecologist immediately referred her to a local neurologist. After taking a family history and listening to her symptoms, the neurologist had Emily take an MRI scan. She was almost 99% sure she knew what Emily had: MS.

It was classic.

Once Emily got over her shock, surprise hit: How could this happen? She had always lived a healthy life. She exercised and ate her vegetables. "What's going on here???" she cried when her neurologist gave her the news.

She was sure that Emily had had a first occurrence years ago: some slight dizziness . . . a sudden loss of balance . . . tremors or tingling in her arms or legs . . . numbness on one side of her body. Subtle symptoms that went away in a few weeks, seemingly harmless by themselves, but together: a definite reason to see a doctor.

The neurologist immediately put Emily on an intervenous steroid treatment. After five days, it would be followed with another 10 days of steroids in pill form. This would help reduce the inflammation of the myelin sheaths that were affected; it would quiet the immediate symptoms.

Although the disease-modifying drugs would have been more effective if Emily had started taking them when she first had her early symptoms years before, they could still do the job now. They could still help the progression of her MS as well as keep additional episodes at bay.

Today, Emily is still taking care of herself, eating right and exercising. She has added stress reduction to her routine with yoga classes and meditating. She takes her MS medication without fail and she has learned to live with her disease. She has continued her job in the publishing company and, although she has had a few more episodes, her level of functioning has not deteriorated.

And, oh yes, Emily calls her doctor or nurse whenever she feels the need—and she always urges others who were just as stubborn as she once was to reach for help if they need it.

Emily's story is, unfortunately, a typical one for MS patients. Oftentimes, people don't report their early symptoms. The symptoms don't seem too bad or dangerous; they don't want to disturb their doctor. They tell themselves it's nothing; the symptoms will go away by themselves. All good excuses and perhaps valid. But here's a lesson we all have to learn:

The only way to rule out the possibility of MS is to see your doctor at the first sign of any of these symptoms. Early, aggressive treatment can make all the difference in the progression of your disease.

This chapter is designed to help you recognize those early symptoms. If you experience any of these, call your doctor for an appointment. It's not frivolous. It's not intrusive. It's smart.

EARLY SYMPTOM ALERTS

The following symptoms have all been found in people with MS. They are considered early symptoms because they may be the first manifestation of MS. They are frequently part of the early relapses and remissions in a person's disease. They are the "red flags" you need to see your doctor about if you experience one or more. *(We will be going over specific treatments for the most common symptoms of MS in Part 4 of this book.)*

Red Flag #1: "Pins and Needles" or Sensory Disturbance

You are all familiar with that tingling feeling that occurs when your foot or hand has fallen "asleep". When you haven't used your hands or feet for a while, circulation stops flowing or a nerve gets temporarily compressed, and you might even experience numbness—followed by those pins and needles once you've begun to "shake that body."

In multiple sclerosis, however, the numbness and tingly feeling isn't from a hand or foot falling asleep. It's not caused by circulation problems; it is caused by lesions in the central nervous system. Nor does the pins-and-needles sensation occur when you haven't moved for hours. You may suddenly feel a sensory disturbance on your skin—or you may gradually feel the "pins and needles" getting stronger. Whatever the onset, this symptom can crop up at any time and usually fades within a short period of time.

You might feel a tingling or a numbness on one whole side of your body and face, or, if a spinal cord lesion is involved, your arms and legs on both sides. A feeling of pressure or a "squeezing" sensation around your chest or from your belly button down may also indicate spinal cord lesions.

Many people with early MS symptoms frequently describe unusual sensations on their skin, such as burning, creepy-crawly itchiness, or supersensitivity to touch. These odd feelings are called dysesthesias and may be accompanied by pain.

The most creative description of this early symptom comes from a patient who described it as if she had a wet fish wrapped around her waist.

Although this "pins-and-needles-like" symptom is one of the most common seen in MS, it can be difficult to diagnose. The feeling might be so subtle that you barely notice it. Even a neurologist may have difficulty detecting any abnormality when you are experiencing a feeling without displaying any physical evidence.

Red Flag #2: "A Crick in the Neck" or Lhermitte's Sign

Many people forget to tell their doctor about this one because it happens quickly—and quickly goes away. As a person with MS bends her head and neck forward in a "ducking" motion, she may feel an electric shock sensation travel down her back. Lhermitte's sign is due to inflammation of the myelin in the spinal cord; the "short circuit"-like feeling comes from stretching the neck and irritating the inflamed myelin.

Lhermitte's does not automatically equal MS. This symptom is also seen in older adults who have arthritis in their necks—which narrows the spinal canal.

Red Flag #3: "Weak in the Knees" or Weakness in the Extremities

Because MS attacks the insulation that keeps the central nervous system protected and efficient, it makes sense that many of its early symptoms will involve sensory disturbances. It also makes sense that motor function efficiency will be disturbed; you might not feel as strong when you try to lift a grocery bag or when you try to open a jar. Weakness in the extremities can vary from mild to severe; it can involve only one arm or one leg or all four extremities—depending on where the lesions lie in your nervous system. In a study done at the University of California in 1999, 31% of MS patients had some form of muscle weakness when first diagnosed.

Red Flag #4: "I'm All Thumbs" or Clumsiness

If MS lesions have developed in your cerebellum or its connections, it's very possible that your coordination will be affected. You may find yourself dropping things or bumping into furniture. You may also experience a tremor in your hands or feet. Speech, too, can be affected. During an episode of MS, you might slur your words—due to the loss of control of the voluntary muscles that control articulation: your mouth, jaw, or tongue. This condition is called dysarthria.

Red Flag #5: "Doing the Drunk" or Gait Problems

This symptom, too, is a result of MS lesions in the cerebellum or the neural pathways leading up it. Called gait ataxia, this symptom involves the voluntary muscles you use to walk one step in front of the other. Instead, you may become unsteady on your feet; your walking pattern might mimic that of a very drunk or dizzy person.

Red Flag #6: "Pain in the Eye" or Optic Neuritis

Like Emily, the MS patient we described at the beginning of this chapter, you may experience optic neuritis as your first or early MS symptom. Here, the myelin inflammation and subsequent lesions attack the optic nerve, which sits right behind the eyeball. Because the optic nerve cannot now efficiently conduct visual messages to the brain, certain symptoms of optic neuritis may crop up: You might find your vision dimming or your color vision affected. You might also feel a searing pain or ache in or behind your eye. Optic neuritis is one of the most common signs of MS. In the same University of North California study we mentioned earlier, 29% of the MS patients had an episode of optic neuritis—

and 53% of all people with optic neuritis developed MS within 5 years.

Red Flag #7: "Double Trouble" or Vision Problems

Your MS eyesight problems are not always the result of a lesion in the optic nerve. Inflammation and lesion damage in your brainstem may cause different symptoms involving your sight.

Vision problems have many names: diplopia, unilateral internuclear ophthalmoplegia (INO), and nystagmus (jiggling, rapid movements of the eyes). But no matter what you call it, your eye coordination is off. Ordinarily, your brainstem connects one eye with the other so that when you look to the left, both eyes move and, when you look to the right, both eyes move again. When lesions occur in your brainstem area, they affect this primal, coordinated, choreographed movement. Your eyes are no longer in sync, and you may see double or your vision may seem like it jumps.

Red Flag #8: "I Need a Nap" or Fatigue

This one's big, the most common symptom that crops up in MS patients. Indeed, 90% of patients with MS experience this extreme tiredness at one time or another.

And it's serious. If you are tired, you cannot get through your day. You become lethargic, inefficient, and, possibly, depressed. We normally feel good after a workout or a solid day of work, but people with MS do not have the same good feeling. Because of the inflammation and erosion of the myelin sheath, messages are not efficiently conducted through the CNS; the electrical message cannot get through rapidly. Instead of feeling good, people with MS may feel extreme fatigue after a workout—and they are not able to do as much work as they had before. Sleepiness means tired—and tired translates into a lack of energy. Add weakened muscles and cognitive problems from lesions in the brain, and the fatigue becomes much more than a need to take a nap. *(You will find energy management techniques to battle fatigue in Part 4.)*

HOT AND BOTHERED

People who have fatigue due to MS lesions need to use more than sunblock when they go outside on a hot summer day. MS makes them extremely sensitive to heat. Why? Because as core body temperature rises from the heat, nerves become even less efficient. If you have MS and want to work in your garden, do so on cloudy, cool days—and take lots of breaks in an air-conditioned room. Large hats, neck wraps with ice cubes, and even cooling vests can make a big difference. Don't forget to try a cool shower before and after exercise. Cool drinks will also help.

Red Flag #9: "Primal Attack" or Bladder and Bowel Dysfunction

There are so many things we take for granted: getting dressed, tying our shoes, brushing our teeth—and going to the bathroom when we feel the need.

For people with MS lesions in their spinal cord pathways, it is a different story. People with MS can very well develop bladder and bowel problems.

This is especially true in the later progression of the disease, but, in five percent of people with MS, bladder dysfunction is one of the very first symptoms to crop up: The need to urinate becomes urgent and may become very real and very embarrassing. Ultimately, bladder dysfunction can result in incontinence or, when the bladder never completely empties, a urinary tract infection. (Fifty percent of men who have this MS symptom also suffer from sexual problems, especially impotence.)

Bowel dysfunction is even more common: 60% of all MS patients suffer constipation. Although this problem can be the result of certain medications or a low-fiber diet, it can also be a significant sign of MS lesions in the spinal cord.

Unfortunately, incontinence and constipation most definitely affect a person's quality of life. People who have bladder or bowel problems—regardless of whether or not it

---

GOING BY THE NUMBERS

As reported in Multiple Sclerosis: A Reappraisal, *a study done by Dr. D. McAlpine and his colleagues in London found that early MS symptoms, seen individually or in combination with each other, break down as follows:*

40% of people with MS: weakness in the arms or legs
22%: optic neuritis
21%: sensory disturbances
12%: double vision
5%: dizziness (gait ataxia) and vomiting
5%: bladder dysfunction

stems from MS—retreat from society. Their self-esteem is markedly diminished. *(You'll find strategic treatments for bladder and bowel management in Part 4.)*

Now that you know the early symptoms of MS, you need to know what can happen later, down the road, as—and if— your disease progresses. You'll find details on these later symptoms of MS next.

MAKING A TURN:
LATER SYMPTOMS OF MS

*I know multiple sclerosis isn't a life-threatening dis-
ease, but it sure has changed my life—in some ways
even for the better. Sure, I have to use a stroller to get
around. And I can get really moody at times. But, on
the other hand, my MS got me to think about things
more. I try to meet challenges with courage. And I
appreciate everything I have. I know this sounds
funny, but I feel stronger than I ever have in my life.*

—A 53-year-old female television executive
with secondary-progressive MS

- Jonas couldn't stand the pain. He had gotten used to the
  idea that he couldn't walk. He understood that he
  couldn't open jars or carry heavy bundles. He coped:
  Instead of running, he did water exercises. He read
  books. He began using adaptive devices to help him get
  around in his law firm office and his home. But the pain
  was something else entirely. Sometimes it was his
  lower back. Sometimes it was from his spastic muscles.
  With the help of his doctor and his rehabilitation team,
  Jonas could manage the pain most of the time. And he
  thanked God that he lived in a world where MS could
  be managed.
- Marion had once been a schoolteacher; she taught history in the local high school. But that was before her
  MS symptoms began to worsen—and crop up more.
  For her the cognitive problems were the worst: She

hated the fact that sometimes she couldn't remember a word or read a passage in a book. She hated the fact that she couldn't always remember what someone had just said. Although the disease-modifying drugs hadn't yet been created when Marion was diagnosed with MS, she is on one of them now and it's been helping her. Her rehabilitation speech and occupational therapists she meets with three times a week at her local rehabilitation center also helps keep Marion's condition stable. She can now read the latest Patricia Cornwall mystery like everyone else.

- Alicia's MS problem was spasticity. Her left hand clenched, and her left arm curled inward; she couldn't move it. As hard as she tried, her left arm stayed where it was. Alicia was glad she had her electric scooter; she was able to use it to get out of her apartment, do errands, and make meals for her family of five. But when the spasticity set in, she was helpless. Luckily, she'd gone to a rehabilitation facility that specialized in MS. Her physical therapist helped her strengthen her muscles on a daily basis; she also took prescribed pills which eased her spastic muscles and she could now more easily get around. Life felt good to Alicia. Very good. She knew solid, reliable help was only a short drive away.

- Marcus had been a real *bon vivant* in his early years. He'd partied hard and went out with a lot of women. When he settled down with his wife, his sex life only improved. They had a good marriage and an active one. But when Marcus developed MS symptoms in his early forties, things changed. At first, the change was subtle: some weakness, a little difficulty in seeing. But each time Marcus had a relapse, the symptoms got progressively worse. Now his MS had affected his sex life. He was impotent—along with half the men who get MS. That didn't console him. He just wanted to be able to enjoy himself again! But MS specialists at his rehabilitation center were able to help there, too. Marcus was able to talk frankly with his doctor and his therapists; they, in turn, suggested medication and ways to improve intimacy between him and his wife. Lo and behold . . . they worked!

These people have more in common than having MS. They have all experienced symptoms that can occur as the disease progresses. The more lesions that crop up, the more disabling the symptoms. But, as these short examples also show, even disabling symptoms can be treated successfully.

Here, in this chapter, you'll discover in detail what the later symptoms of MS are—and in Part 4, you'll learn how to treat them all.

BETTER NEVER THAN LATE

Ideally, everyone who is diagnosed with MS is treated early and aggressively with disease-modifying therapy and rehabilitation therapy. Ideally, too, MS symptoms disappear after a few weeks or months—never to return.

But we live in a less-than-ideal world and, unfortunately, most of the time MS becomes progressively worse. New symptoms crop up, and some of them can be debilitating even with treatment.

Let's go over the later symptoms, the critical "Red Flashes" of MS, now:

Red Flash #1: "What Was I Saying?" or Cognitive Decline

As more and more lesions pop up in the brain, its tissue is eventually damaged—to the point where memory problems may occur or organizational skills may be lost. The total number of lesions correlates directly with the amount of intellectual functioning lost. Thus, in the early stages of MS, cognitive decline will either be non-existent—or so subtle that it's barely perceptible. But as more lesions build up in the brain, problems become much more apparent. Approximately 40% of MS patients lose some sort of intellectual function during the course of the disease, usually:

- Short-term memory loss (forgetting something that was just told to you, or within a few hours)
- Difficulty in managing certain tasks (such as some complex executive functions and decision-making)
- Confusion
- Loss of attention span
- Inability to concentrate

Unfortunately, it makes sense that MS will affect your intellect. After all, the inflammation involves your brain and damages its pathways. But the good news is that early treatment may reduce cognitive decline. The disease-modifying drugs may slow down or completely halt the inflammation

---

The Best Treatment Plan: Think Early, Think Aggressive!

and the appearance of new lesions. This means less risk of losing your intellectual prowess.

Red Flash #2: "Helpless and Hopeless" or Depression

Which comes first, the chicken or the egg? The depression that comes from damaged brain connections or the depression that comes from knowing you have MS?

The answer is probably a combination of both: sadness caused by damaged connections in the brain and sadness caused by the reality that, yes, you have a serious neurological disease. Nor is your depression an isolated incident: 70% of all MS patients suffer from depression, especially in the later stages. In fact, it's the second most common MS symptom after fatigue—and it is found more often in MS than any other neurological disease.

It might not sound as bad as, say, bladder problems or double vision, but depression, even by itself, can be a "silent" disabler. It can rob MS patients of their self-esteem, their motivation, and their hope—and affect their treatment's success. In fact, patients who have MS are 7.5 times more likely to have suicidal thoughts than the general population.

You'll read more about treating depression in Part 4, but, for now, know that it can be stopped in its tracks with today's very effective antidepressants—in conjunction with therapeutic counseling.

Red Flash #3: "I'm in the Mood . . ." or Emotional Lability

There's a myth about MS that we would like to dispel right now: People who have MS are not always happy—even though they may laugh at unusual times. People with MS are *sometimes* happy—and sometimes not, just like everyone else. The same dysfunctional pathways in the brain that create depression can also create mood swings and inappropriate laughter. When signals to the brain go haywire, unusual things can happen, like abruptly crying in the middle of a conversation or laughing all the way through a movie.

Again, as with depression or cognitive decline, the more lesions in the brain, the more changes in behavior—and the more mood swings that seemingly "take over" a person's life.

Fortunately, this problem is successfully managed by medication for many people.

Red Flash #4: "Like a Spinning Top" or Vertigo

The classic Alfred Hitchcock movie *Vertigo* dealt with the psychological dizziness some people have when they look down from a great height. To add suspense, Hitchcock had his phobic main character chased up a spiraling staircase in a high tower—and then forced to look down at the ground from the very top.

Unlike the dizziness experienced by this Hitchcock character, the symptom of vertigo that some MS patients experience is not psychologically based. It is a very real and physical result of lesions in the brainstem. Although approximately five percent of people experience vertigo, or dizziness, at the onset of MS, most of the people with MS experience this as a late symptom—40 to 50% in fact. In some cases, the vertigo is accompanied by vomiting.

Red Flash #5: "Not Tonight" or Sexual Dysfunction

Another very real symptom of MS in its later stages is sexual dysfunction. The spinal nerves that supply our genitals are exceedingly sensitive to disease or injury—whether it's caused by a traumatic fall or by the inflammation and damage in the spinal cord that defines MS. Men may become impotent, having either erectile or ejaculation problems. Women may experience the loss of sensation or anorgasmia (the inability to have an orgasm).

Sexual problems may also be a result of *other* MS symptoms, such as fatigue, spasticity, bladder or bowel problems, cognitive impairments, pain, tremors, or sensory problems. You can also have sexual problems as a result of certain medications you are taking for your MS. All these very real physical problems can inhibit sexual pleasure and intimacy.

Further, the depression and emotional stress of having MS can stop a person from enjoying sex. The psychological, social, and cultural implications of having MS can put up barriers that seduction cannot break.

The good news is that more and more healthcare professionals are beginning to recognize sexual dysfunction as a very real problem in MS. They have become educated and can help patients learn about various treatments, adaptive devices, and strategies. *(You'll read all about this in Part 4.)*

Red Flash #6: "What Did You Say?" or Paroxysmal Dysarthria

Think of stammering or stuttering and you'll have an idea what paroxysmal dysarthria is all about. It is an MS symptom that involves speech. Paroxysmal means sharp, sudden, intermittent spasms. The dysarthria in its name means a slurring of speech or an eccentric, erratic pattern of speech. Paroxysmal dysarthria can come and go at any time; it can last for only minutes or for hours at a time. Although we don't understand the patterns these spasms take, we do know that, unlike other motor skills affected by MS, paroxysmal dysarthria is not caused by damage and inflammation in the spinal cord. It is caused by MS lesions in the corticobular area of the brain—either in the nerves leading to the part of the cortex that controls speech motor skills, in the reticular formation, or in pathways relaying sensory perceptions from the mouth and throat area to the brain. *(See Chapter 3 for in-depth information on these and other parts of the brain.)*

Red Flash #7: "That's Hard to Swallow" or Dysphagia

There are many conditions and accidents that can cause problems with your ability to swallow. Spinal cord injury, brain injury, or stroke can make the usually automatic swallowing action difficult—if not impossible. Because it can affect self-esteem and the ability to be independent, rehabilitation teams first focus on getting patients to regain this ability to swallow.

In multiple sclerosis, dysphagia, or difficulty in swallowing, may be caused by a combination of factors. The problem may be weakened throat muscles, tight spastic muscles, difficulty with coordinating the act of swallowing—or all three.

Red Flash #8: "I Can't Move!" or Trouble Walking

When the spinal cord nerves become inflamed and develop lesions, it can, of course, affect your mobility. A limb may feel very weak, or become paralyzed; one side of the body or both arms and/or legs could be affected.

Unfortunately, as we've mentioned earlier, 50% of people who have MS will eventually need help in getting around, either with a cane, a scooter, or a wheelchair. *(We believe this number will drop as more and more MS patients are diagnosed more efficiently and treated more quickly and aggressively with disease-modifying medication.)*

Further, any spasticity *(see Red Flash #9)* you have may be too severe for you to walk, or your lack of coordination may have progressed to the point where walking isn't safe. Many times it is the sum of all the accumulated lesions and disability that tips the scale.

WHEN A WINK IS NOT A BLINK

Another symptom of MS involves the nerves in the face. Tic douloureux, or trigeminal neuralgia, is a condition that makes you feel as if electrical shocks are shooting through your face. You might feel a burning sensation or an intense sharp pain. Only five percent of MS patients develop this symptom, but it can be very painful. Several medications are highly effective in controlling this pain. (See Part 4 for an in-depth look at pain management.)

Red Flash #9: "The Curling Cry" or Spasticity

When MS inflammation or lesions appear in the CNS, they can cause weakness (quadraparesis)—as you've already discovered. But these same lesions can go the opposite way— they can create muscles that are not only weak but too stiff.

When a muscle contracts, the motion is a reflex action, an automatic response. But when your spinal cord nerves are damaged by MS lesions, they cannot receive a message from the brain that tells them to move that elbow back down, to uncurl that hand, to bend that straightened knee, to flex those pointed toes. Muscles stay tight, right where they are, and contracted. The reflex action is frozen. If they remain in a rigid, straight form, you are in the midst of an *extensor spasm*. If they remain bent or curled, you are having a *flexor spasm*.

Spasticity can also lead to contractures, a condition in which the tissues surrounding your muscles and joints become so tight that you cannot even use the muscles that are working, that are getting the nerve messages to relax.

There are many conditions that can create spasticity's characteristic too-tight muscles: Cerebral palsy, spinal cord injury, brain injury, and stroke, to name a few. In MS the spasticity can arise from lesions in the brain, in the spinal cord, or in both areas. The degree of spasticity and the frequency of spasms may vary at first with the activity of the disease. Later on, spasticity may be a permanent feature of your disease.

When an MS person has spasticity, she will walk more slowly than other people. He might drag one foot or have both feet move across each other like a scissors. She might need crutches. He might use a scooter to get around. Sometimes a leg will lock up; sometimes the muscle will weaken.

The good news for spasticity is that there are many treatment plans available to release and relieve its pain. Spasticity doesn't always have to be disabling—as you will discover in Part 4.

HYPO HYPE

Another symptom, much less common than spasticity but similar to it, is called hypotonia. It is the opposite of spasticity. Here, muscle tone is decreased or completely absent; a leg or arm may be limp like a rag-doll. There isn't enough tone left to support useful movements.

Red Flash #10: "Pain, Pain, Go Away" or Migraine Headaches and Other MS Pain

No one likes pain, whether it emanates from a sprained ankle or a stomachache. Although MS is thought of more as a disabling disease than a painful one, more than half the people with MS suffer from some kind of pain. In one study, 55% of the MS patients had pain at least once during the course of their disease; another 48% had chronic pain that didn't go away.

Pain with MS makes sense: nerve endings are askew; messages to and from the brain are not getting through accurately; insulation of nerve fibers is raw and inflamed; and sensory perceptions may be heightened. People with MS may be highly sensitive to pain.

The pain associated with MS can either be as a result of the disease—or as a result of one of its symptoms. Pain is pain, but there are different types when it comes to MS:

- *Paroxysmal pain* is a sharp, intermittent pain that may occur from spasticity, brain, or spinal cord inflammation. People sometimes experience a burning sensation or a shooting electrical shock. Tic Douloureux is a form of paroxysmal pain. So is the sharp pain of suddenly spastic muscles.

- *Facial neuralgia* affects the fifth cranial nerve; nerve disturbances along this pathway can create that intense sharp paroxysmal pain at the jaw, cheeks, lips, even forehead, eye sockets, and mouth.
- *Paroxysmal limb pain* can occur suddenly in the arms and legs. This limb pain is experienced as either a burning or itching feeling, or as an ache that lasts for seconds or minutes.
- *Migraine headaches* are another form of paroxysmal pain. Although the connection between MS and headaches is not clear, research shows that people with MS get more headaches than the general population. Sometimes a person may experience an *aura* before the migraine hits. This is a visual type of migraine headache, in which you see either sparkling lights, zigzag lines, or bands of rainbow color. The visuals end just as the migraine begins. (Seeing auras or having a migraine headache does not mean you have multiple sclerosis. In fact, migraine is so common that at least 15% of the population experiences migraine headaches.)

Chronic pain is different; it does not come and go. It is defined as pain that stays at least six months or longer. There are two types of chronic pain that are common in patients with MS:

- *Dysesthetic Extremity Pain* occurs most often in people who have little disability or symptoms. It is a form of nerve sensitivity because of myelin damage. Dysesthetic extremity pain usually involves the legs and the feet, but it can sometimes affect the arms and the torso as well. Some people describe this constant pain as a prickling sensation, a feeling of tightness, or a dull, aching burn. This pain is usually experienced after a bout of exercise, or when the weather changes or gets hot. It is also felt more often at bedtime than during the day.

- *Chronic back pain* is a result of the physical stress that MS can put on your bones, muscles, and joints as you move about. It can also occur because you sit or stand too long. It can also be a result of compensation; using stronger muscles to help weaker ones can put a lot of stress on the body.

Pain can also come from some of your MS symptoms: a urinary tract infection due to bladder problems, a headache caused by double vision, a bruise or a cut from gait imbalances.

Yes, pain is very real—but there are effective medicines, smart strategies, and wonderful adaptive equipment that can help ease the worst of it. *(You'll read more about pain management in Part 4.)*

These, then, are the symptoms you may experience, either singly or in combination with each other, maybe more than once—or maybe not at all.

As you now know, multiple sclerosis is unpredictable. You may have one episode and go about your life a long time before you feel its symptoms again. On the other hand, you may have many relapses, each one more debilitating than the one before.

Let's explore this unpredictable terrain a bit more—and learn about the four basic "roads" MS usually takes.

CHAPTER SIX

THE DIFFERENT ROADS MS CAN TAKE: A CLINICAL COURSE

I had my first bout of MS a year ago. I had tremors, tingling in my fingers, and it was difficult to walk. But most of the symptoms went away in a few weeks. Soon I was back on my feet like nothing had happened. I ignored the problem—until it worsened again 3 months later and didn't get any better. My doctor told me I had the kind of MS that is progressive. I am slowly getting worse, but fortunately rehab and the drug mitoxantrone have been a big help.

–A 38-year-old male corporate manager
with primary-progressive multiple sclerosis

Eva was a good doctor. She cared about her patients and she always called them as a follow-up to make sure they weren't in pain. As a small town internist, she was always busy. If she wasn't treating Mrs. Costern for her arthritis, she was treating Billy for the cut knee he got in the playground. Old, young, chronically sick, occasionally under the weather, serious, and benign—Eva saw them all and took care of them as best she could.

When Eva wasn't playing doctor, she was playing wife and mother—to 3-year-old twins. Sure, she had help, but she liked to spend as much time with her family as possible.

Eva had a good, productive life. She couldn't remember being happier. Her husband, a contractor, had just made her a surprise 39th birthday party. All her friends were there, as well as her medical staff and her family. The twins had made adorable cards that already had a permanent place on the refrigerator door.

And then the face pain hit: sharp pain that made her stop in her tracks. She actually had to come home from the office and lie down—something she never, ever did. She took sinus medicine, but the pain continued. She told herself that she was too young for trigeminal neuralgia, or electric shock-like pain in your face. *(See Chapter Five for more information on this condition.)*

But it wasn't just the face pain. She also noticed weakness in her right hand, a tingly sensation in her toes, and dizziness.

As a doctor, Eva knew that something was wrong with her nervous system. She didn't want to think it was MS. But, deep in her heart, she knew that all the signs pointed to the disease.

Eva made an appointment with a neurologist, a colleague of hers in the next town. She had an MRI performed. The news wasn't great: Eva had MS and there were decisions to make about her life.

Fortunately, Eva's doctor believed in the new disease-modifying drugs called the "ABC + Rs" (so named for the first letter of each particular drug). He immediately put her on steroids to take care of the current symptoms, and then pre-scribed one of the disease-modifying medications to help avoid future relapses—or, at the very least, help make them less severe.

Routines had to change at home and at the office. Eva con-tinued to practice medicine, but she brought in a younger doc-tor, fresh out of his hospital residency, to help her out. She hired a full-time housekeeper to help with the family chores. She explained what was happening very carefully to her children. She told them that sometimes she wouldn't be able to play with them. Sometimes she would need quiet time. The twins understood that sometimes their mother was sick and they respected the new household "rules." Eva's husband was extremely supportive; he helped around the house as well.

Eva was lucky. She had savings and her husband made a good living. They wouldn't feel a financial pinch too much. She was knowledgeable about the disease; she knew how to take care of herself and how to prevent bladder problems and back pain.

Others weren't so fortunate and Eva took on a second job: she became a spokesperson for her local chapter of the National Multiple Sclerosis Society. She led a support group and helped answer questions.

Eva still loved her life. She had her husband, her children, and a satisfying career. Perhaps she needed a scooter to get around. Perhaps she took longer to make a decision. Perhaps she sometimes got depressed. No matter: life was here and now and it was good.

Eva's story is not a typical one. Most people feel they've been assaulted when they first learn they have MS. It affects their personal lives, their business lives, every facet of every day. It's no wonder that many people do not tell anyone about their disease, hoping it will just go away; they are afraid of losing their jobs, their friends, even their closest relationships.

MS is still a mystery in many ways. And it is still extremely misunderstood by the general public. But we have been able to pinpoint four different clinical courses that MS may take. Hopefully, the explanations that follow will help solve your MS "mystery".

RAREFIED AIR: BENIGN MS

In the best of all possible worlds, you will have one or two episodes—and never have another one again for the rest of your life. These episodes usually consist of either a numbing sensation or temporary vision problems, usually optic neuritis. Because these symptoms flare up infrequently, many people do not seek out their doctor—but that is a mistake. Less than five percent of people are fortunate enough to have benign MS.

SOLVING THE MYSTERY: THE BIG FOUR

The majority of people who have multiple sclerosis fall into one of four categories, one of four clinical courses that have been recognized by scientists who specialize in MS research all over the globe:

Mystery Solution #1: Ups and Downs
Relapsing-Remitting MS (RRMS)

Mary Beth, a 48-year-old stockbroker, had one episode of MS when she was a teenager; she had had a bout of double vision that went away within two days. She'd forgotten about it until she had a second episode in her 30s: vision problems and a tingling feeling in her right hand that also disappeared within a few days. But she was smart enough to see a neurologist at that point: It wasn't normal to have tingling that didn't go away when she shook her hand "awake." The neurologist told her she had MS and, at that point, she remembered the double vision she had had in college. She had a third episode, a year later. Once more she had vision problems and a tingling feeling in her right hand for two weeks. Mary Beth will most likely have another episode someday, but she refuses to live her life "waiting for the other shoe to drop." The times between each episode are symptom-free, and the injections she takes conscientiously help keep her that way.

Approximately 70% of all people who have MS fit into this category at some time throughout their lives—and 90% of all MS patients, even those who currently have progressive symptoms, begin here, with RRMS.

Like living every day, sometimes joyful, other times sad, this is an on-again/off-again type of MS that is categorized by very clearly defined episodes (the relapse phase) followed by periods of months or even years when there are either no symptoms at all, or at least no new symptoms (remission phase).

During a remitting cycle, people with MS may feel completely fine—with all their MS symptoms gone as if they'd never occurred. For others, the MS symptoms linger; they don't get worse during their remission, but they might be left with lingering symptoms: vision problems, a sensitivity to heat, or a slightly wobbly walk.

Each subsequent episode leaves most people with residual disability. The flare-ups are acute and more debilitating. During the remission phase, these more debilitating symptoms may disappear, linger in a more benign form, or remain for good. But you should not get worse during a true remission; it is only during the relapse stage that your symptoms worsen. During remission, your symptoms tend to remain at a plateau. However, that does not mean that changes are not taking place in your brain. That is why early treatment is so important.

So where's the mystery? In knowing when the next relapse is going to occur. Some people are in a remission for years; others only a few months. We cannot chart a predictable course for RRMS, but we do know that beginning a regimen of a disease-modifying drug at the very first onset of symptoms can reduce the frequency of relapses and their seriousness.

**To repeat, over and over again:
Treat early and treat aggressively.**

Mystery Solution #2: Changing Gears
Secondary Progressive MS (SPMS)

Elisa was a 45-year-old mother and grandmother—and she had more energy than her two grandchildren put together. To someone outside the family, Elisa would seem to be the prototype for living a healthy life: She exercised, and she ate lots of fruits and vegetables. But, in reality, Elisa had MS. She'd been diagnosed in her 20s, before effective medications existed. She'd been put on heavy doses of steroids and her dizziness, tremors, and numb feeling went away. She'd had four other episodes since then. The next two episodes were as mild as her first one: some dizziness, tremors, and a numb feeling in her fingers and toes. In between, her symptoms practically disappeared. But the last two episodes were a different story: Elisa not only had the "usual" symptoms, but she found that she could barely walk. She was very, very tired. Her MS symptoms were more severe. But, after each acute flare-up, she was left with a bit more disabling symptoms; they didn't go away, but they weren't as severe. Elisa could walk, but she sometimes lost her balance; she was weaker and needed to take frequent naps. She dreaded the next acute attack: She knew it would create even more disabling symptoms. She hoped the medication she was using would put off that next relapse and slow the progression of her disease.

It happens. Things don't always work out the way we wish. Sudden surprises can hit and change everything. That's what happens with secondary progressive MS. It starts out as an RRMS but eventually something causes it to change, and it grows progressively worse. Approximately 80–90% of all people with RRMS evolve into secondary-progressive MS.

Secondary-progressive MS travels a circuitous route; it can involve minor remissions and relapses, plateaus and acute flare-ups—at any given time.

If your relapsing-remitting MS has turned into secondary-progressive MS, there is hope. No, you can't erase the symptoms you have, but they can be treated—with good rehabilitation, strategies for managing daily life, and medicines that truly work.

Mystery Solution #3: A Slippery Slide
Primary Progressive MS (PPMS)

June, a 45-year-old English professor, has learned to live with her MS, a disease that had created havoc in her central nervous system since her late thirties. She has never experienced a remission; nor does she have acute attacks. Instead, she has slowly become more disabled as time passes: going from a walker to a scooter to a wheelchair. Her cognitive abilities have declined; she is more confused and she has difficulty paying attention. She has lived with her disease half of her life and she has learned to accept it— thanks to physical therapy at her nearby rehabilitation center, a clinical psychologist to help her handle her emotions, and a support group where she can share her story with others who are in the same situation.

Why do some people start out with a more severe disease course than others? We don't know. Ten percent of people start out with debilitating symptoms and never have remissions; their multiple sclerosis continues to erode their quality of life. There are medications today that can help and there are specific treatments to ease the effects of each symptom.

THE CLUES

True, we still cannot say with absolute certainty why some people have an easier time between attacks—or why some people have one or two attacks and never experience MS symptoms again. Nor do we know why some people "switch" from relapsing-remitting MS to secondary-progressive MS. Nor can we cannot predict the future—but we can offer some clues:

- *Most people who have MS "burn out."* They simply stop having attacks. Their symptoms stabilize at some point and never worsen.
- *Women who are pregnant usually do not experience relapses.* They have healthy pregnancies. There is something about the hormonal changes during pregnancy that affects the course of the disease. Researchers are exploring this as an area of potential treatment.
- *More women than men get MS,* but they have a more favorable outcome when they do.
- *People who have symptoms that involve sensory problems, including optic neuritis, have a better prognosis* than people who have cerebellar or motor problems such as weakness and lack of coordination.
- *Most people develop MS between the ages of 20 and 50 years.*
- *Although we don't know which virus, if any, to blame, the Epstein-Barr virus* is currently number one on the list.
- *MS has nothing to do with trauma or tragic accidents.* It cannot be caused by trauma—nor do traumatic events trigger a relapse.
- *MS cannot be worsened from flu or hepatitis shots.* So make sure you get the protection you need!
- *Hot weather can make all MS symptoms worse.* People with MS have a high degree of sensitivity when it comes to heat. The combination of body heat and faulty electrical insulation around their nerves makes their systems slow down. We call this thermosensitivity.

SEXUAL TENSIONS

Women not only get MS twice as much as men, but they are more at risk for all autoimmune system diseases, including lupus and rheumatoid arthritis.

We do know that estrogen may affect the way our immune systems respond. A study has found that 70% of women have more intense MS symptoms right before their periods.

Progesterone, which is produced cyclically and during pregnancy, can decrease immune response— which may explain why there are few MS relapses when a woman is pregnant: her immune system is quiet; it is not "attacking itself."

Women who have MS can take birth control pills (which contain estrogen). In fact, one study found that the pills might have had a protective effect similar to pregnancy while women with MS were taking them.

There is research currently being done on whether sex hormones can be used as therapeutic agents in halting the severity of MS.

We know now the mysterious ways of multiple sclerosis. You know the way the disease can develop and you know the symptoms—both early and late. It's time now to make a diagnosis: Do you have MS or not?

CHAPTER SEVEN

MAKING THE DIAGNOSIS: YOU HAVE MS

Having multiple sclerosis is not the end of the world.
It's just a different beginning.

—A 42-year-old father of three
who has learned to live with his MS

They brought me into a dressing room where I was told to change into a hospital gown that tied in the back. I was told to take off any jewelry, my watch, and anything, like a hearing aid or a metal dental bridge, that might disrupt its magnetic field. I was scared—not only of the fear that I might have MS, but by the diagnostic test itself. MRI. It sounds like a song or a symbol, not a test that involves a magnetic field!

I'm in the room now and lying down on some kind of futuristic bed; it's all white. Everything in the room is white. There's a humming noise in the background and it's very cold. The nurses tell me to relax but it's hard. I feel like I've just entered a science-fiction movie.

The radiology technician pats my shoulder and smiles. It won't take too long. He proceeds to tell me what will happen—that the MRI uses magnetic energy and radio frequencies to enable a scanner to transmit information about my brain, brainstem, and spinal cord to a computer in an outside room. The information is translated into extremely accurate pictures of my central nervous system.

Okay, okay. I have no idea what he is talking about. I just want it to be over. It sounds much too complicated.

He then goes on to tell me I will hear odd, clanking, sometimes loud noises when the magnetic energy is being used.

I'm still not sure about the whole thing. I'm still nervous, but I think I can handle loud, weird noises. After all, I'm not a kid! But then he asks me if I'm claustrophobic. Huh?

I hear him over my loud, anxious thoughts. 'If you are at all claustrophobic, we can give you a tranquilizer to calm your nerves.' I want to shut out his voice.

Am I claustrophobic? I can't think of any situation where I might have felt trapped—at least not until this moment. I whisper no. I am so scared that I can't make my voice any louder.

"I'm going to give you an injection of a chemical dye now," he continues. "It's called a contrast agent and it will enhance the images of the MRI. It won't hurt."

Famous last words. "Ouch! Okay. . . ." It's done. A chemical is now coursing through my body and I'm about to enter a tunnel.

The nurses put a shower cap on my head. Are they going to watch me take a shower now? They're still smiling, as if they are all in on a private joke that I don't get. Stop it! I'm getting paranoid.

Paranoid, huh? Then why is everyone leaving? . . . Oh, I see them. They are in a cubicle, behind a glass wall. The technician smiles and gives me the "thumbs up" sign.

I try to smile back. The bed starts to move. I am moving. Slowly. Slowly. Directly under this huge white, noisy machine. I look up. The machine feels like it is moving down towards me. I remember Edgar Allen Poe's *The Pit and the Pendulum*. The pendulum coming closer and closer. . . .

"Eek!" I screech. I should have taken the guy up on the tranquilizer.

"Eek," I screech again, but my heart's not in it. Let's just get this over with. . . .

The loud, humming noise is intermittent, but I don't feel any pain. Nothing. I am beginning to relax. It's like I'm in a gigantic cocoon. If it doesn't get any worse than this, I'll be okay.

I close my eyes and—just like that!—I'm rolled away from the machine. It didn't feel like an hour.

"You did great. Thanks!" the assistant says, coming back into the room. "We got some great images."

I smile, trooper that I am.

As I get up to leave, I realize how important this test is. This will help my doctor to make an accurate diagnosis and decide if I need treatment. I can get on with my life.

Do I dare say it? I'm glad I had this test. It was nothing! Just wish it wasn't so darn cold . . .

This scenario is one that is currently going on in hospitals and imaging centers across the country. MRIs are an important tool for diagnosing many neurological conditions—from tumors and stroke to MS. MRIs are particularly crucial for helping to determine multiple sclerosis because it can show if there are multiple lesions—even though the patient seemingly had only one episode.

But there are other tests that are used to help diagnose multiple sclerosis. Some of these tests are used to rule out other conditions. Others may be used before an MRI is ordered. And still others may be used to confirm an MRI's findings, especially if the lesions are not clear-cut.

This chapter explains the different tools and tests neurologists use before making a confirmed diagnosis of MS.

PRE-MRI: NOT SO LONG AGO

Just 30 years ago, doctors had to be more observers than active participants. They would have patients take the "hot bathtub test." A tub was filled with warm water and, after a thorough examination, a patient literally took a bath. After getting out of the tub, the neurologist examined the patient again to see if there were any neurological changes. Because MS can make a person sensitive to heat, any negative changes suggested the patient had the disease.

They also gave even greater importance to optic neuritis. Because 50% of people with MS started out with this condition, doctors used it as a "test" evaluating the Uthoff Phenomenon (named for the doctor who first described how symptoms worsen—or are even caused by—exposure to heat). After thorough examinations, patients performed some form of intense exercise. They would then be checked to see if their vision, or other MS symptom, grew worse.

Communication is always crucial—in life and in diagnosing a disease. But it is even more important when it comes to MS because early symptoms can be so very subtle. And, in the days before the MRI, communication was the only way to dig up clues.

TALK TO ME

Taking a complete medical history is still vital, even in these days of routine MRIs. It remains the first line of inquiry.

A DIAGNOSIS OF EXCLUSION

Whether years ago or just yesterday, the diagnostic process for any neurologist is akin to solving a crime. Other conditions have to be ruled out before MS can be pinpointed. The more diseases that you don't have, the easier it can be to know what you do have. This process is called a differential diagnosis and involves the medical history, neurological examination, radiology testing, and lab work.

Once your internist or ophthalmologist decides your symptoms show more than simply blurred vision due to eye strain or the need for a change in eyeglass prescription, a neurologist will be called in.

On your very first visit, the neurologist will ask you many detailed questions, including:

- When did you notice your first symptoms? What were you doing? What made you take stock of them?
- Why did the symptoms feel strange?
- Have your symptoms progressed? How?
- Do you remember any time in the past that you might have experienced similar symptoms?
- How often do these symptoms appear? Do they go away and come back—or are they constant?
- Are you in any pain?

Your neurologist will also ask you general questions about your health and your family's health. He will ask:

- Do you have any already-diagnosed conditions, such as high blood pressure, arthritis, or asthma? Does anyone in your immediate family have these conditions?
- Does anyone in your family have any neurological problems?
- Do you have any allergies and, if so, what are they?
- Do you exercise? Have you noticed any physical changes when you are exercising now?
- How are your moods lately? Have there been any sudden mood changes?
- How is your appetite? What kind of foods do you normally eat?
- Are you experiencing any bladder or bowel changes?
- Do you smoke or drink?
- Have you had any memory problems?
- Would you say you are an energetic person? Have there been any changes in your energy level?

Probing further, your neurologist will also ask you about your place of birth, where you lived when you were a child, even about your work environment. Anything can offer up a clue. Do you have a neurological condition? Is it MS?

THE NEUROLOGICAL EXAM

You are not ready for an MRI just yet. After spending time exploring your medical and lifestyle history, the neurologist will perform a series of tests in his office to test your reflexes, your muscle tone, and your eyes. To an outsider,

THE BASICS: WHY A NEUROLOGIST?

A neurologist is a medical doctor who has had three or more extra years studying the diseases of the nervous system. She diagnoses and treats any disease of the brain, spinal cord, and the peripheral nervous system.

A neurosurgeon also specializes in diseases of the nervous system, but he also performs operations that need to be done.

Since multiple sclerosis is a disease of the nervous system that usually requires medical treatment without surgery, people who may have MS will be referred by their family doctor to a neurologist.

these tests can look like "ding-dong school" at recess time, but, in reality, these seemingly simple tests can reveal a great deal about you.

The neurologist will start with the head and work down to your feet. The exam will include:

- *An eye exam.* The neurologist will look in each eye to get a good view of your optic nerve—is it pale or swollen? Using fingers or a pencil, he will check to see that you have full peripheral and central vision. He will also observe the eyelids to see if one of them is drooping; he will ask you to look to the right, then the left, to determine your eye coordination.

- *A hearing and speaking test.* Engaging you in a regular conversation, the neurologist will notice if you have trouble hearing or if you are slurring any words. He may use a tuning fork to check your hearing.
- *Cranial Nerves Testing.* You will be asked to close your eyes, smile, stick out your tongue and even try to recognize various odors with your eyes closed. All these seemingly strange exercises test your cranial nerves.
- *The Walk.* Your neurologist will watch you walk, to a scale, down the hall, or to pick up a folder; he wants to see if you have a gait problem, if you are wobbling or dizzy, or if one foot drags slightly. Can you walk as if you were on a tightrope with one foot directly in front of the other?
- *Muscle tone and strength testing.* To check your strength, you might be asked to push against your doctor's arm; each individual set of muscles can be tested quickly through squeezing, pushing and pulling. To test your muscle tone, he will note whether your arms and legs move freely or have any increased resistance. (Spasticity, for example, would make it difficult to straighten out a flexed arm or bend a straightened knee.)
- *Reflexes.* That little rubber hammer can tell your doctor a good deal. When the neurologist taps on your arms, knees and ankles with his hammer, your body usually responds with a jerky motion. The neurologist can then observe if your reflexes are normal, under, or overactive. These can be sensitive signs of neurologic disease.

- *The Babinski or extensor plantar reflex test.* This classic neurological test tells volumes with a simple stroke on the sole of your foot—with a key or any type of blunt instrument. In healthy people, the big toe will automatically point down. If the central nervous system tract running from the cortex to the spinal cord (called the corticospinal tract) is damaged, the big toe will point up.
- *Cerebellar and Coordination Testing.* When your doctor asks you to touch your finger to your nose, she is not playing "Simon Says." She is watching your hand to see if there is a subtle side-to-side tremor that could indicate cerebellar problems. You may be asked to tap your hand or foot quickly to see if the movement is smooth and regular.
- *Sensory perception tests.* These tests examine all our senses—from spatial perception to the sense of touch, from temperature perception to the ability to feel. Your neurologist determines your sensory damage, if any, with tests that range from having you stand up and close your eyes (to see if you can maintain your balance without sight) to placing a vibrating tuning fork to various points on your body (to determine if you can tell when the motion stops), from pricking your skin with a pin (to see if you can feel in different parts of your body) to checking light touch with a stroke of his finger.
- *Memory tests.* Your doctor may ask you to memorize three or four simple words and repeat them back to him five minutes later. He may ask you the day of the week and the year or spell "world" backwards. These tests are not flashbacks to grade school; they can help determine your mental acuity.

In addition to testing specific neurological functions, your doctor will also give you a thorough physical exam, including an examination of your skull to look for any abnormalities; he will also check your blood pressure and listen to your neck and heart beat to see if your symptoms point to a different disease.

THE BOTTOM LINE: THE MRI AND OTHER LABORATORY TESTS

Your doctor now has a good sense of you: your symptoms, your family history, your medical past and present. He has done a thorough neurological examination and has determined where there is damage to your central nervous system. He can now determine a probable diagnosis: multiple sclerosis.

But to remove all doubt, he needs to actually see your brain, your brainstem, and your spinal cord. He needs an MRI.

The Diagnostic King: The MRI

The exact name for it is Magnetic Resonance Imaging—and almost everyone suspected of having MS will have one. Because an MRI shows the structure of the entire central nervous system in stark detail, it is by far the most useful tool for finding multiple lesions—and where they are located.

Like the woman at the beginning of this chapter, an MRI can feel imposing, scary, a sci-fi apparatus. But, also like that same woman, once you know what the MRI entails, the fear goes away. To that end, here's a brief description of what it is and how it works:

An MRI involves a combination of computer technology and physics. An MRI uses radio frequencies and a powerful magnet to chart electrical charges as they surge through the brain, the brain stem, and the spinal cord. It then converts these charges into computerized, highly detailed pictures of the brain. These pictures clearly and efficiently display lesions in the central nervous system.

Because MRIs so clearly show multiple lesions, a doctor may not have to wait until you've had multiple episodes to make a diagnosis. He can have an MRI done if you display any possible symptoms—and see almost immediately whether there is more than one lesion in the brain or spinal cord. Depending on the number of lesions and the location of each one, she may or may not feel comfortable making a definite diagnosis of MS.

To help detail any inflammation as well as show active lesions that are currently at work on the myelin and its nerve cells, a harmless chemical contrast agent will sometimes be injected into a person before the MRI. The one used most often is Gd++, or gadolinium, and it was the agent that was most likely used in the example at the beginning of this chapter.

As much as we rely on an MRI to make a multiple sclerosis diagnosis, it is not an "exact science." Things can change in the brain without our being aware of them. Serial MRIs, for example, have been performed on patients with absolutely no complaints. The MRI scans on these patients reveal that, from month to month, lesions can disappear, pop back up, and then disappear again. The message: MS can be very active in the brain without our knowing it!

Lesions that are there for good—and which cannot be helped with disease-modifying drugs—show up on the MRI scan as black holes in the white matter. These holes represent destroyed axons, which cannot be repaired.

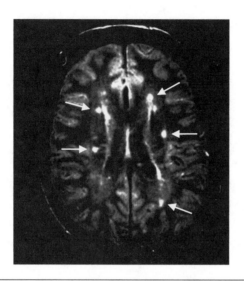

An MRI scan of the brain of a person who was just diagnosed with MS, demonstrating a mild amount of multiple Bright T2 lesions (arrows) on both sides of the brain in the periventricular region. This is early in the disease course and the ventricles are normal in size. (Images courtesy of Rohit Bakshi, MD, Assoc. Prof. Neurology, University of Buffalo, State University of New York)

How do you determine the extent of MS—and whether it is really there? If the MRI shows multiple lesions and you have had multiple episodes involving the central nervous system, it is safe to assume you have MS.

If the MRI shows multiple lesions but you had only one episode, your doctor may still feel comfortable making a diagnosis of MS and start treatment right away.

But sometimes a diagnosis is not so clear. Things change in the brain all the time; your symptoms might be too subtle to notice; lesions might not be appear distinct enough on a particular scan. In these situations, other testing is needed to confirm an MS diagnosis. These tests include:

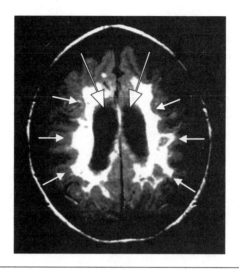

An MRI scan of the brain of a person who has had MS for many years. There are now large confluent Bright T2 lesions (small arrows) surrounding the ventricles. The ventricles are enlarged and there is evidence of cerebral atrophy (large arrows). (Images courtesy of Rohit Bakshi, MD, Assoc. Prof. Neurology, University of Buffalo, State University of New York)

The Power Behind the Throne: Evoked Potentials

This has nothing to do with living up to your potential—or appearing on one of those "We'll Make You a Star" type of shows. Evoked potentials are a series of specific tests that look at various parts of the nervous system—by measuring the way your nervous system reacts to specific visual, auditory, and sensory stimuli.

Electrodes are attached to various spots on the scalp, neck, and limbs; visual, hearing and feeling stimuli are then used to activate nerve signals and a machine records how long it takes for the evoked nerves' message to reach the brain. The rate of speed is an indication of damage in the brain's sensory pathways; the slower the transmission, the greater the damage. About 65% of people who have definite MS will show abnormalities in the passageways.

The type of evoked potential used in diagnosing MS is the *Visual Evoked Potentials (VEP)*. Here, electricity is supplied to the back of the head (where vision is controlled) while the patient watches a checkerboard on a screen. If the speed at which the optic nerve conducts the electricity up to the brain is slower than it should be, there is an abnormality present.

VEPs are used predominantly when the diagnosis is in question and your doctor is trying to find additional lesions in your central nervous system.

The Second in Command: A CT Scan
An MRI is always the first choice in making a diagnosis of MS. But because of its strong magnetic force, it is very sensitive to any pieces of metal that are in its path. That's the reason why you must take off all your jewelry—and dentures— before the test.

But there are pieces of metal that you can't remove: shrapnel from an old war wound, a pacemaker, a metal plate—these can all affect the accuracy of an MRI. They can also be moved and turned around during the test—causing the potential for harm. A pacemaker, for example, that is pushed out of position or altered can have serious implications for your heart.

In these cases, a CT Scan will be given. Although less accurate than an MRI, the CT Scan (short for Computerized Axial Tomography Scan) is a highly accurate and powerful X-Ray. The large donut-shaped machine that you lie in is like a powerful camera that takes pictures of your brain in slices. It photographically "peels away" layers of tissue.

Although not as accurate, a CT Scan can be very helpful for those patients who are unable to tolerate or have a MRI performed.

The Old Regimen: Spinal Tap

Yes, there is a very funny movie about a rock band called *Spinal Tap*. This spinal tap, however, has nothing to do with entertainment.

Basically, after numbing your skin to take away any pain, a thin needle is inserted in your lower back and a few teaspoons of spinal fluid, the liquid that bathes and supports the spinal column and the brain, is drawn out. The spinal fluid is then examined for signs of an overactive immune system using two specific tests, an oligoclonal bands myelin basic protein test that closely examines your CNS, and another test that details your immune system's activity—an IgG synthesis index.

Although these tests are not specific enough to diagnose MS on their own, when combined with the right signs and symptoms, they help confirm its diagnosis. Although a spinal tap (or lumbar puncture, as it is sometimes called) was commonplace in the past, many neurologists today feel comfortable not performing it when the MRI and clinical picture strongly confirm a positive diagnosis of MS.

The diagnosis has come in: You have multiple sclerosis. The tests show there is no doubt. But it is not the end of the world. Today there are amazing new medications that can help control your MS. There are also proven treatments to improve your *specific* symptoms as well as your quality of life.

The journey is not over—not by a long shot. In the next section you'll discover some of the new treatments for MS that are available.

PART THREE

THE WINDING ROAD

CHAPTER EIGHT

POWERFUL MEDICINE AT WORK: ACUTE CARE AND THE "ABC + R" DISEASE-MODIFYING DRUGS

I am so happy I have MS now—and not ten years ago. Today, thanks to the MRI, my doctor was able to diagnose my condition in its early stages. He immediately put me on one of the disease-modifying drugs—and my MS has stopped progressing. My symptoms have eased and I am living a completely normal life. I feel blessed—and grateful I live in an era of so many medical advances!

—A 48-year-old female librarian
with relapsing-remitting MS

Elliot would do his mother proud. At 38 he was a highly successful psychiatrist with groundbreaking research published in international journals, several mainstream books under his belt, and a successful practice in the heart of beautiful San Francisco.

You would never know he had multiple sclerosis; he sometimes forgot himself.

He'd had his first episode in medical school and decided that he'd best go into a specialty that would accommodate any unforeseen future disability. Psychiatry was perfect; he would be able to sit and not walk from room to room all day. He also had a fascination with the human mind and had done some work on brain chemistry while in school.

The first ten years went well. He married and had two children; he moved his practice from a room in his home to an office in Mission Hill. He had a view of the Golden Gate Bridge as it glimmered at dusk. He had a few relapses, but nothing that couldn't be managed with intravenous steroids. He knew when the numbness would begin, when his speech would get slightly slurred, when his left hand would begin to shake. Before the symptoms got worse, he'd see his neurologist and have his relapse taken care of immediately. The intravenous steroids always did the job.

Elliot had read about the new ABC + R drugs in one of his journals. They sounded promising, compelling. He decided to enroll in one of the first studies of these drugs in the United States. He had an excellent response to one of these specific disease-modifying therapies and had no relapses. He was able to work, drive his car, play golf with his friends, and travel to Europe with his family. He'd almost forgotten that he had MS.

Unfortunately, in the last year he had not one, but two relapses—and they left him more disabled each time. He became fatigued and could barely keep his head up past noon. He needed to use a cart to play golf, no longer able to enjoy walking on the expansive green. He used a scooter more and more often to get around, in stores, in the mall, whenever he had to do things outside the house. He found himself banging into things, the chair in his office, the kitchen table, the television set. And, to add insult to injury, he became impotent.

Obviously, the drugs had stopped working after all these years. But he had to do something: His relapsing-remitting MS was turning into secondary-progressive and steadily growing worse.

When Elliot had a follow-up MRI, he was shocked to see how many new lesions there were in the white matter of his brain. He became scared. What if he couldn't practice anymore? What if he couldn't enjoy traveling and spending time with his family? What if his cognitive abilities started to decline?

But there was hope. A drug normally used for chemotherapy called Navantrone® (mitoxantrone) had recently produced excellent results when given for secondary-progressive MS. Since Elliot's neurologist wasn't sure if he was "officially" in the secondary-progressive stage, he didn't want to stop his particular ABC + R drug treatment. Instead, he added the Navantrone® to Elliot's medical regimen. He would be given an intravenous infusion of the drug once every three months; time would tell if it was effective.

Meanwhile, Elliot is doing what he has to do: scaling back his office hours, meeting with a physical therapist to work out an exercise routine, and working with an occupational therapist to find strategies to conserve his energy.

The signs look good, and Elliot is hopeful. He can still practice part-time, he can still play golf, and, the best yet, he can spend quality time with his wife and kids.

As Elliot's story proves, medicine does work. Multiple sclerosis symptoms can be alleviated during acute attacks and, even better, reduced with disease-modifying drugs.

We've come a long way from the days when neurologists diagnosed, then said adios! There was nothing they could do, and people with MS had to live their lives wondering when the next attack would hit.

No more.

In this chapter, we will discuss both the drugs used during an attack—and the new disease-modifying drugs that have quite literally changed thousands of lives.

GOLDEN GOALS

"First, do no harm!" That is the goal of any health care professional. And, as with any chronic disease, this motto goes further: to stop the pain, the inflammation, or any symptom that may be causing a disability. But MS is complicated—and other treatment goals are necessary:

- *Reduce relapses.* Thanks to the "ABC + R" disease-modifying drugs this can be a reality.
- *Decrease severity and duration of relapses when they occur.* Treating patients with a steroid regimen helps reduce the inflammation that is causing the relapse.
- *Recognize, treat, and decrease disabling symptoms.* In addition to disease-modifying medication, a patient with MS should be in a rehabilitation program where any symptom that hinders a good quality of life can be treated.
- *Slow down or prevent remitting-relapsing MS from becoming secondary-progressive.* Like Elliot in our example at the beginning of this chapter, a combination of disease-modifying drugs may help do this.

ATTACK! ATTACK!

If you have an MS episode, be it a relapse or the first one, the prime object is to stop it—as quickly as possible. Neurologists today have several options—all of them successful for most people with MS.

Steroids Do More Than Make Big Muscles

Slight numbness might not be enough to warrant heavy doses of steroids, but if your symptoms are serious enough to affect your ability to function, your neurologist may use a 500–1000 mg. intravenous (IV) drip of methylprednisolone (IVMP) every day for three to five days; the drip can be done by a nurse at home or on an outpatient basis in your doctor's office. If your symptoms are serious enough, you might receive your IV in a rehabilitation hospital—where you can get therapy in addition to your medication for a double bang! After the three to five days on an IV, you will most likely take prednisone pills for ten days, starting with a high dose and slowly decreasing it each day so you are finished by day ten.

Steroids work: They stop the inflammation that causes your symptoms. They shorten the duration of your episode and accelerate recovery. But they don't alter your MS course and they don't prevent another episode from occurring when you least expect it. One study of 457 MS patients with optic neuritis found that they had a significantly quicker and more effective rate of recovery when they had IV methylprednisolone therapy; this was especially true for those patients whose optic neuritis symptoms were the worst. But six months later, the group that had had the IVMP had no more advantage than the group that hadn't been given steroids. Both had the same visual acuity; both were equally susceptible to another attack.

Another steroid, dexamethasone, has been found to have the same results as IVMP, but the final results are not yet in. Because it is less expensive than IVMP in other countries, it is used more overseas.

Although NSAIDS (Non-steroid anti-inflammatory drugs) such as ibuprofen (Advil® or Motrin®) and naproxen (Aleve®), as well as other common agents like acetaminiphen (Tylenol®) and aspirin, work well for muscle aches and pains, they don't have any effect on the actual course of MS.

THE BLOOD-BRAIN BARRIER

Call this The Great Wall . . . The Last Defense . . . The King's Guard . . . the blood-brain barrier is that important. It is a biological shield that ordinarily prevents circulating substances in the blood from getting into the spinal cord and brain. In MS, however, our antibodies are able to pass through this barrier—and they immediately start attacking our nerves. But sometimes it's important for certain chemicals to get in: the medicines we need to get healthy. When scientists create a new medicine, they have to make sure their final product can seep through the blood-brain barrier.

From Me to Me: Plasma Transfers
Perhaps steroids never worked for you—or they just don't work as well as they used to. Whatever the reason, when steroids don't work on an MS patient, there are alternatives. One of these is plasmapheresis, or plasma exchange. Here, blood is actually taken from you and put through a machine that takes out and "cleans" the white blood cells (and the immune system cells that have become your enemy) and

returns spanking clean blood back into your body. Presumably the white blood cells that have been attacking your myelin sheaths have disappeared—and your symptoms will also disappear. The process may be repeated several times.

The problem? Plasma transfers must be done in a hospital setting, they are very expensive, and they work only 40% of the time.

LESS FAVORABLE MS PROGNOSIS

- *Older at onset*
- *Male*
- *More severe episodes at onset*
- *More lesions seen on initial MRI*
- *High relapse rate, especially within the first two years*
- *Early prominent motor or cerebral function impairment*

The Protector: Immunotherapy

Let's say your body has not responded well to steroids; your symptoms are still acute and disabling. There is another choice besides plasmapheresis and it is called IV immunoglobulin, or IVIG for short.

Here, instead of steroids being dripped into your body from an IV, rich, thick, pooled immunoglobulin is put into your bloodstream. These energetic, new Igs will presumably attack the confused white blood cell antibodies; they will attack your once upon a time immune system friends, destroy them, and, in turn, destroy your acute symptoms. Your relapse will hopefully disappear.

We don't know exactly why IVIG works as well as it does; nor do we know the exact dosage to administer. But the important thing is we do know it works for some people with MS.

The only drawbacks? IVIG is very expensive (approximately $5000–$10,000 per infusion!), and not every health plan covers it. If steroids work for you, they should be the relapse medication of choice.

BETTER MS PROGNOSIS

- *MS begins at a younger age*
- *Female*
- *Normal initial MRI*
- *Complete recovery after first episode—and a long interval before the second*
- *Very few relapses*
- *Little disability two and four years after your diagnosis*

A STEADY COURSE: KNOW YOUR ABCs and Your R

Okay, you now know what to do if you have a relapse. But what about in between relapses? Are you supposed to just wait and watch, a passive victim of your disease?

A resounding no! Today there are the disease-modifying drugs, the ABC + Rs of multiple sclerosis management, that have changed the way we look at MS. They have enabled people with MS to live healthier lives with less disability. They have helped prevent their disease from progressing more rapidly. They can also reduce relapses—and increase the time in between episodes.

Although this sounds too good to be true, it is all possible—thanks to years and years of cutting edge study, research, and clinical research. The result? The disease-modifying ABC + R drugs: **A**vonex®, **B**etaseron®, **C**opaxone®, and **R**ebif® (which was added to the "ABC" list in 2002). And, for worsening relapsing MS and secondary-progressive MS, the Food and Drug Administration has added a fifth letter: "N"—for Novantrone®.

The fact that these medicines exist to change and modify the course of your disease is extraordinary. But what is more extraordinary—and unfortunate—is that only 40% of patients who would benefit from them actually take them!

Sadly, many people who have their first episode of MS are reluctant to start a course of medical treatment. They want to wait until they've had a second relapse—and many of their doctors concur. But it's most likely wishful thinking to believe your MS is benign. There's such a small group of people who have benign MS that the odds are against you. And the next relapse might be more serious than the first. Damage to your myelin sheaths and the axons of your nerve cells could be much worse—and irreversible—the second time around.

Remember: Treat early and treat aggressively!

A IS FOR AVONEX®

The scientific name for Avonex® is interferon beta–1a and it became available in May 1996 from the pharmaceutical firm Biogen. Although we don't know exactly how Avonex® does its good work, the important thing is that it does—by blocking interferon gamma, the immune system chemical that may be responsible for your body's attack on itself. By blocking interferon gamma, it can regulate and slow your body's immune response against itself, in particular, myelin and the cells that make it.

Going by the Numbers

Clinical studies done at the State University of New York at Buffalo, the Cleveland Clinic Foundation, the Good Samaritan Hospital and Medical Center in Portland, and the Walter Reed Army Medical Center and Georgetown University, both in Washington, D.C. have found that Avonex®:

- Decreases the frequency of MS attacks by 32% over a two-year period.
- Delays the likelihood of MS getting worse (going from a single episode to a multiple one) by 44% over a three-year period.
- Decreases the amount of disability accumulated from relapse to relapse.
- Actually reduces asymptomatic, or "silent", lesions (which can still create a loss of brain tissue and cells) by 91%—and reduces lesions that cause visible neurological symptoms by 52% within a two-year period.
- Decreases the worsening of cognitive impairment by 47%.

How to Use It

Avonex® is made using DNA technology—via an amino acid (the building blocks of DNA) structure identical to the natural interferon our bodies make. It is a weekly intramuscular medicine, which means that it is injected into either the large arm or leg muscles once a week. By injecting the medicine, it quickly goes into your bloodstream and starts to work. The usual dose is 30 mcg.

Avonex® comes prepackaged with a one-month supply; each week's "dose pack" contains everything you need to administer your injection: a single-use vial of Avonex®, a single-use vial of Diluent, a vial access pin, a syringe, needle, alcohol wipes, a gauze pad, and an adhesive bandage. Ideally, Avonex® should be kept refrigerated, but it can be stored at room temperature for up to 30 days (in case you are traveling). Instructions are easy to understand and your physician or nurse will show you step-by-step how it is administered. A health care provider can also teach a family member to give it to you if you find it difficult to give yourself an injection. There is also Avonex® support on line at www.msActiveSource.com. You can also reach ActiveSource by phone at 1-800-456-2255. The organization offers information, personal injection training, administration support to help get you started, and, through their Avonex® Alliance, provides free extra needles and syringes for emergencies.

Side Effects—And How to Treat Them

The side effects of Avonex® are manageable, and may include:

- Flu-like symptoms
- Muscle aches

- Fever
- Chills

Headaches, pain, and weakness were about the same for the Avonex®-taking group and the control group (who took nothing). The side effects usually go away within the first 24 hours and decrease as time goes by. Side effects can also be kept to a minimum if you start with a lower dosage and build up to the optimal one.

To help you manage any flu-like symptoms that may occur, your doctor may recommend taking an analgesic, such as acetaminophen (Tylenol®) or ibuprofen (Advil®). You can also time your weekly injections so that you administer them right before you go to bed; you'll sleep through the worst of it! Studies have also found that antidepressants such as Prozac® can keep flu-like symptoms at bay.

Because Avonex® is an interferon drug, it may affect your liver. Periodic blood tests will check that your liver enzymes stay in balance. Avonex® may also depress your white blood cell count which can also be detected by regular blood tests.

The only people who should avoid Avonex® are women who are or are considering getting pregnant; people who have a history of seizure disorders; and people who are currently being treated for depression.

The Advantage
Why Avonex®? Because the medicine:

- Has shown good results with people who have relapsing-remitting MS.
- Decreases severity and frequency of episodes.

THE INFO ON INTERFERON:
A VERY SIMPLE PRIMER

There's a lot of talk about interferon medications in helping many diseases, including hepatitis, AIDs, and now multiple sclerosis. But what exactly is an interferon? Its definition is complicated and whole books are written about its structure and its effects, but, because we talk about interferons when we talk about the disease-modifying drugs, it's important to have some sense of what it is. Very simply put, interferons (IFNs) are small protein molecules called cytokines that are naturally produced by immune system cells (see chapter 3). These IFNs (cytokines) are created in response to several "intruders," especially those that are a virus—which is a good thing. These IFN molecules are powerful antiviral soldiers divided into separate "regiments" by their different amino acid structures: either alpha type 1, beta type 1, or gamma type 2. In MS, for reasons that are unclear, there is less of the interferon gamma produced in your cerebrospinal fluid. When you take an interferon medication you give your body a strong reinforcement of the other antiviral interferons, alpha and beta, that for some reason stimulates the production of gamma. By changing the IFN equation, immune cells may be stopped from attacking your nerve cell's myelin which, in turn, may halt the progression of many viral-induced autoimmune system diseases—like MS.

- Is convenient. It only needs to be taken once a week.
- Has shown to be effective in reducing cognitive impairment.
- Reduces the number of new MRI lesions.
- Has shown only a 4% injection-site reaction (burning, itching, or swelling) in several clinical studies.

Financial Aid

Avonex®, as with all the interferon drugs, does not come cheap. At this time, prices for Avonex® are approximately $13,000 per year. Fortunately, there are organizations, in addition to your individual health plan, that can help pay for your medication. Avonex®'s MS ActiveSource and the Avonex® Reimbursement Hotline can answer your questions about medicare, medicaid, and other state and federal programs and see if you are eligible. (The annual income cut-off point for reimbursement is currently $60,000.)

B IS FOR BETASERON®

The "B" drug of choice is Betaseron®, the first interferon medication that was approved by the Food and Drug Administration. Betaseron®, produced by the pharmaceutical company Berlex, differs only slightly from Avonex®. It is an interferon beta–1b. This means that it is an interferon medication with a very similar molecular structure to Avonex®. The difference? One amino acid: cysteine is substituted for one called serine. More than 126,000 people worldwide have been treated with Betaseron® since it was first introduced in December 1993.

Going by the Numbers

The groundbreaking clinical study proving that interferon beta-1b (Betaseron®) was effective in treating relapsing-remitting MS appeared in 1993 in *Neurology*. This study and others demonstrated that Betaseron®:

- Reduces the frequency of MS attacks by 30% over a five-year period.
- Reduces the severity of attacks by 50%.
- Decreases disability progression in people with relapsing-remitting MS.
- Reduces the rate of relapses in people with secondary-progression MS by 30%.
- Decreases the number of total MS lesion areas in the central nervous system by 104% over a two-year period.
- Decreases the appearance of new MS lesions by 80% over a two-year period.

How You Use It

Betaseron® is given by subcutaneous injection every other day. This means that the injection you give yourself involves a small, thin needle that goes just under the surface of the skin. If you have trouble giving yourself the injection, an auto-injector (a spring-loaded pen-like device) will make it easier to give yourself just the right dose. When you start on Betaseron® therapy, you receive a free in-person training with a nurse who will help you learn how to mix and inject the drug, as well as answer any questions that may come up.

The usual dosage of Betaseron® is .25 mg, averaging to 28 million IU per week. You can receive a full 100-day supply of materials—including 50 small needles you'll use for your Betaseron® dose, 50 large needles you'll use for your Diluent (a sodium chloride solution that mixes with your medication), a container for throwing away your used needles, and 200 alcohol swabs—by calling Betaseron®'s MS Pathways at 1-800-788-1467. Your pharmacist will supply your vials of Betaseron® and your Diluent. Betaseron® may be kept at room temperature for added convenience.

Betaseron® also provides additional sources of support: an introductory video, "Voices of Experience"; a 24-hour hotline staffed by registered nurses specializing in MS; a Personal Patient Assistant who becomes your personalized contact every time you call; and reimbursement counselors who act as advocates with insurers. You can contact any of these services by calling the Betaseron®'s MS Pathways hotline at the above number or by visiting Berlex's MS Resource Center at www.Betaseron.com.

Side Effects—And How to Treat Them

The main side effect of Betaseron® can be soreness, itchiness or redness at the injection site one or two days later. To decrease skin reactions:

- Ice the injection site before administrating the shot.
- Apply an anesthetic cream, such as Elamax® or Emla® before you give yourself an injection, or use an anti-inflammatory cream like 1% hydrocortisone cream afterwards. *(Note: Dermatologists are concerned about long-term use of hydrocortisone creams.)*
- Rotate your injection sites. Don't use the same spot every time. (Injection reactions occur less frequently in areas with more fat, such as your stomach or buttocks.)

- Gently rub the injection site for a few minutes after you've given yourself your shot. This will help distribute the medicine under your skin.
- Allow your Betaseron® to reach room temperature before using.

As with Avonex®, another side effect may be flu-like symptoms, such as chills, fever, sweating, and muscle aches. To decrease your chances of feeling sick, take some ibuprofen such as Motrin®, or acetaminophen such as Tylenol®, a half-hour before injecting your Betaseron®. It also helps to give yourself the injection right before you go to bed so the flu-like effects, if they occur at all, will happen while you are asleep. Keeping some Tylenol® or Motrin® by your bed can help, just in case you wake up in the middle of the night feeling sick.

DEPRESSION COMPRESSION

Five percent of the people who take interferons get depressed. Since depression is a symptom of MS in and of itself, this is a hard one to call. If you are suffering from depression as a part of your MS symptoms, you should be under your doctor's care. And if you find yourself feeling depressed while taking any of the interferon drugs, talk to your doctor. (Note: The "C" drug Copaxone® does not have depression as a side effect.)

To keep side effects to a minimum, your doctor may start you on a partial dose of Betaseron®, increasing it gradually over the first month.

The Advantage

Why Betaseron®? Because the medicine:

- Has shown good results with people who have relapsing-remitting MS.
- Decreases severity and frequency of episodes.
- Decreases the formation of new MRI lesions.
- Decreases cognitive deterioration.
- Can be given subcutaenously with an Auto-injector.

Financial Aid

At this time, prices for Betaseron® are approximately $13,000 per year—about the same as Avonex®. Fortunately, there are organizations, in addition to your individual health plan, that can help pay for your medication. Betaseron®'s MS Pathways and the Betaseron® Foundation (whom you can contact at www.Betaseronfoundation.org) can answer your questions about Medicare and Medicaid, as well as other state and federal programs, to see if you are eligible. (The program is designed to help people whose income is approximately 3.5 times the federal poverty cutoff line. This means that the cutoff is approximately the same as it is for Avonex®: $60,000.)

C IS FOR COPAXONE®

Unlike the other ABC + R drugs, Copaxone® is not an interferon medication. Instead of having a natural amino acid structure, Copaxone® is a synthetic chemical compound called a polymer which is made from a combination of four amino acids: L-glutamic acid, L-alanine, L-lysine, and L-tryosine. No two combinations are the same; each person receives a different ratio of these four amino acids with each dose. This drug may work by mimicking the structure of myelin so that your T-cells attack the Copaxone®—instead of your nerve cells. Although it takes longer for Copaxone® to take effect than Avonex® or Betaseron®, it may be a good choice for people who have trouble taking the interferon medications. Made by Teva Neuroscience, Copaxone® was introduced in this country in December 1996.

Going by the Numbers

Studies published in the *New England Journal of Medicine* in 1987 and *Neurology* in 1995 demonstrated that Copaxone®:

- Decreases acute attacks by 32% over a two-year period.
- Reduces the lesions seen on MRI by 35%.
- May attack the killer T-cells and simulate the production of myelin.
- Produced no increase in disabilities in 78% of relapsing-remitting MS patients over a two-year period.

How to Use It

Copaxone®, like Betaseron® is given by subcutaneous injection just under the skin. You must give yourself an injection every day. Teva Neuroscience has just come out with a pre-mixed syringe (a "mixject" Vial Adapter) to be used with an FDA-approved autoject® injector which does the work for you. The usual dose is 20 mg.

Support from Copaxone® comes from Shared Solutions™, which partners you with an individual nurse/counselor to answer all your questions, as well as injection training by a nurse who will come to your house. Shared Solutions™ also provides a 12-month daily planner to help you keep track of your injections and keep you motivated with information, inspiration, and helpful tips, as well as a quarterly newsletter, *Common Ground*, an introductory video, and a delivery service for your medication, Caremark, which can either deliver your Copaxone® to your house or local pharmacy. You can reach Shared Solutions™ at 1-800-887-8100, 8:00 A.M. to 11:00 P.M., Eastern Standard Time, or on the web at www. sharedsolutions.com.

Initial studies of an oral pill form of Copaxone® showed no benefit, but new studies using a higher dose of the pill are in progress.

Side Effects—And How to Treat Them

Because Copaxone® is given as a subcutaneous injection, the most common side effect are skin reactions at the injection site. These include:

- Redness
- Pain
- Inflammation
- Itching
- A lump at the injection site

Applying an ice pack at the site before injecting, gently rubbing the area after you've given your self the injection, using a topical anesthetic like Elamax® can decrease skin reactions.

Approximately 10% of people can have an immediate post-injection reaction, which may include anxiety, chest tightness, shortness of breath, flushing, and heart palpitations. This reaction lasts only about 15 minutes and seems to occur after several months on Copaxone®; it is also self-limiting—usually disappearing after about seven days of injections.

The Advantage

Why Copaxone®? Because the medicine:

- Decreases severity and frequency of episodes.
- Decreases the number of new MRI lesions.
- Causes no flu-like reactions.
- Subcutaneous injection with an auto-injector available.
- Adds convenience with a pre-filled syringe and accompanying injector.

Financial Aid

At this time, prices for Copaxone® are approximately $13,000 a year. Financial support is available through the Reimbursement Services Group of Shared Solutions™, which also provides medical support and counseling *(see the section "How You Use It" on pages 123–124 for phone number and website information)*. There is no set annual income cut-off and each person's case is evaluated individually.

If all means of possible help have been exhausted, a person is then referred to the Patient Assistance Program run by the National Organization for Rare Disorders for Teva Neuroscience. If you qualify, you can get free or reduced-price supplies of Copaxone® for one year.

R IS FOR REBIF®

These three "ABC" drugs are not your only disease-modifying medication option. Rebif® an interferon beta-1a manufactured by Serono, was approved by the Food and Drug Administration in March 2002. It is made from naturally occurring interferons that are the same as those produced in the human body.

Although its name doesn't fit within the "ABC labeling" of the other disease-modifying drugs, Rebif® is still considered one of them—and is as good a choice as any of the others. In fact, many physicians and professionals now refer to the disease-modifying drugs as "ABC + R."

Going by the Numbers

In France in 1998, Rebif® was found to significantly delay the progression of the disabilities associated with MS; the results were first reported in *The Lancet* in that same year. This two-year PRISM study (so-named for its longer title: **P**revention of **R**elapses and Disability by **I**nterferon beta–1a **S**ubcutaneous **M**S) of 560 relapsing-remitting MS patients found that the drug not only delayed the progression of disabilities, but it also helped prolong the time between relapses and decrease the number of MS lesions.

Another study, called the EVIDENCE (for **EV**idence for Interferon **D**ose-response: **E**uropean–**N**orth American **C**omparative **E**fficacy) involved 677 patients between the ages of 18 and 55 with remitting-relapsing MS. The results after 24 weeks showed that a significant number of the patients taking high dosages of Rebif® did not suffer a relapse. Further, they had a statistically significant reduction in MRI lesions.

How to Use It

Rebif® is available in pre-filled syringes of both 22 mcg and 44 mcg dosages. Like the other disease-modifying drugs, it is administered by injection, in this case a subcutaneous shot given three times a week. It is suggested that patients move slowly to full dosage—beginning with 20% the first two weeks, moving to 50% in the third and fourth weeks, and, if well-tolerated, going to full dose by the fifth week. The injections should be given three times a week at least 48 hours apart. This slow introduction of Rebif® to your system helps reduce side effects.

Rebif® is available in both pre-mixed and powdered forms (which is mixed with a dilutent right before administering) and should be stored in the refrigerator. However, it can remain at room temperature for one month. It is also packaged in ready-to-use, pre-filled syringes with needles already attached to the syringe. Called Rebiject®, this automatic injection system has also been approved by the Food and Drug Administration.

Serono recommends that you take the syringe out of the refrigerator 30 minutes before using; it should be injected at room temperature.

Side Effects—And How to Treat Them

Because Rebif® is given as a subcutaneous injection, the most common side effect are skin reactions at the injection site. These include:

- Redness
- Pain
- Inflammation
- Itching

- A lump at the injection site
- Rare skin breakdown

Applying an ice pack at the site before injecting and gently rubbing the area after you've given yourself the injection can keep irritation at bay. Rotating your injection sites will also help. Applying a topical anesthetic like Elamax® or Emla® can also decrease skin reactions.

Rebif®, also like the other interferons, may cause flu-like symptoms; taking acetaminophen, such as Tylenol®, ibuprofen, such as Motrin®, or plain aspirin will usually reduce the fever and aches and pains associated with the flu.

Because Rebif® is given at higher dosages than the other interferon preparations, it is important that your doctor administer blood tests on a regular basis. High doses of interferon medication may, for a minority of individuals, create liver complications as well as a reduction of white blood cells.

The Advantage

Why Rebif®? Because the medicine:

- Has shown significant good results with people who have relapsing-remitting MS.
- Decreases severity and frequency of episodes.
- Decreases the formation of new MRI lesions.
- Some data suggests that the higher dose given more frequently leads to better results. (However, longer studies and further analysis are needed to confirm this claim.)

Financial Aid

At this time, prices for Rebif® are approximately $17,300 per year. Fortunately, there are organizations, in addition to your individual health plan, that can help pay for your medication. Rebif®'s MS Lifelines is a complimentary service offered to people with multiple sclerosis and their families. You can either

speak to a nurse specialist for injection training or a reimbursement specialist, who can answer your questions about
health insurance, Medicare, Medicaid, and other state and fed-
eral programs and see if you are eligible. Therapy support specialists are also at hand to offer guidance and help in getting
started. The number for MS Lifelines is 1-877-44-REBIF.

A, B, C? Or R? Which drug is right for you? Each of the
ABC + R drugs does its job effectively and successfully. The
decision to take Avonex®, Betaseron®, Copaxone®, or Rebif®
is one that must be made with your doctor—as is the decision
to increase or decrease your dosage, stop it completely, or
even switch from one to another. Some physicians recommend an annual MRI to help in the decision-making process;
it may help see if lesions have disappeared or more have
grown. However, having a yearly MRI is very controversial.
Check with your physician to see what's right for you.

In the end, with so many available choices, only you and
your neurologist can best determine the medical course to
take. This is an area that changes as new data becomes available and it is not the role of this book to pick one type of medication over another. Each company has strong individual
arguments as to why its product is the best and each person
with MS is different. Study the subject and talk to your doctor to decide which is best for you.

And, whatever you decide, always remember: **Treat early
and aggressively—and you just might keep your MS
under control.**

THE OTHER LETTER: N IS FOR NOVANTRONE®

The ABC + R drugs are extremely effective in treating relapsing-remitting multiple sclerosis; all four have been approved
by the Food and Drug Administration. Novantrone® is the
only FDA-approved drug for secondary-progressive MS or

worsening MS. Instead of blocking, mimicking, or slowing down an out-of-kilter immune system, Novantrone® goes after the cells themselves—killing or disrupting the nerve cells that are attacking the spinal cord and the brain.

GOING BY THE NUMBERS

Novantrone®, made by Immunex Corporation, is actually a chemotherapy drug (mitoxantrone) that has been used successfully for ten years in higher doses to treat non-lymphocytic leukemia and prostate cancer. Approved by the FDA for use in multiple sclerosis in 2000, Novantrone® is usually given intravenously every three months. Studies published in the *Journal of Multiple Sclerosis* in 1998 and the *Journal of Neurology, Neurosurgery, and Psychiatry* in 1997 found that Novantrone®:

- Decreases relapse rate by 67%.
- Decreases disability by 61%.
- Reduced new MRI lesions by a significant 85% compared to placebo.
- Is highly effective in treating secondary-progressive MS
- Is effective in treating worsening forms of MS that no longer respond to the ABC + R drugs.

How to Use It

Novantrone® is an immunosuppressive drug given every three months by a 5 to 15-minute long intravenous (by IV through the vein) infusion. It can be done on an outpatient basis in a hospital, clinic, or at a doctor's office. The usual dose is 12mg/m^2 (meter squared).

Doctors prescribe Novantrone® in different ways. Although the good results of Novantrone® were shown when it was given every three months, some neurologists will use it only as a "rescue therapy," giving it to patients with worsening secondary-progressive MS on a once-a-month basis for six months. This regimen provides an aggressive burst of immusuppression medication to "ambush and kill" the cells that are attacking your myelin.

Novantrone® is serious medicine. The highest total cumulative dose a person with MS can receive is 160 mg/m². Anything higher and you may end up with serious damage to your heart. However, the total dose used for MS patients is only 140mg/m². This means that a person getting Novantrone® every three months can easily stay with the therapy for 2 years. *But please note: This is a lifetime dose. Novantrone® can never be used again for any reason.*

While you are on Novantrone®, your heart should be monitored on a regular basis. Although MS studies revealed no cases of congestive heart failure, it can be a very real threat as the dosages of Novantrone® add up. Your doctor can measure your heart's functioning by performing an electrocardiogram and a MUGA (Nuclear Ventriculography)—a test that actually measures how much blood from your heart is pumped out of the left ventricle with each heartbeat. The electrocardiogram and/or MUGA should be done at the onset of your Novantrone® regimen and when the total dose reaches 100mg/m².

The Side Effects—And How to Halt Them

Yes, Novantrone® is indeed powerful medicine—and its side effects are similar to any other chemotherapeutic drug. These include:

- *Nausea* Most nauseous feelings disappear within 24 hours, but to keep them at bay try to avoid eating a few hours before treatment; stay away from sweet, fried, or fatty foods; keep bothersome odors at bay; and lay down for at least two hours after your treatment. You can also stop nausea in its tracks by resting in a chair after eating, breathing deeply, taking antacids, and placing a cool washcloth on your forehead until the feeling passes.

- *Thinning hair* Hair loss on this medication is usually slight and not a major problem. Use mild shampoos and soft hairbrushes. Use a low heat on your hairdryer and avoid perms or hair color while taking Novantrone®.

- *Menstrual disorder* There isn't much you can do to avoid the changes in your period. Sometimes your flow might be heavier, sometimes lighter. Sometimes your period might stop completely (amenorrhea). If you experience this side effect, let your doctor know.

- *Possible infections* Because Novantrone® can lower your white blood cell count (the cells that make up your immune system), you might be more susceptible to infections—especially the first month after each dose. The most common infection for people on Novantrone® is urinary tract infection. If you experience any burning sensation while urinating, pain, or an increased need to urinate, let your doctor know. Further, any infection can cause sore throats, fever, cough, and chills. Let your doctor know if you are not feeling well. Antibiotics can usually take care of any symptoms.

- *Blue Hue* When you take Novantrone®, your urine may turn a blue-green color. The whites of your eyes may also take on a blue tinge. Don't be alarmed! It's completely harmless. It's just the medicine at work. Things will go back to normal within 3 days.

Financial Aid

Health insurance coverage of Novantrone® treatment varies from plan to plan. Before you begin your regimen, check with your insurance company about any restrictions to see if you need to receive any prior authorization before you start.

Your doctor or nurse can also help you through the maze of bureaucracy. Immunex has a special reimbursement hotline available to all healthcare providers to help them with claims, submissions, preauthorizations, and appeals.

COMBOS

The practice of medicine has always been part knowledge—and part instinct. This is even more crucial for MS specialists. They must not only be knowledgeable, compassionate physicians, but they need to add a "dash" of instinct: they need to know when to keep administering particular medi-

---

THE TRAPP FAMILY STINGERS

A study done in 1998 by Dr. Trapp and his colleagues found that even a mild initial episode or a benign MS diagnosis could cause serious damage to nerve cells. The researchers discovered that some of the myelin sheaths covering the axons of the cells actually broke—beyond repair. It's not just damage when you don't treat early and aggressively—it may be irreversible.

cines at the same doses—or when to mix a variety of compounds for the best outcome.

There has been modest success reported when ABC + R drugs have been used with immunosuppressive drugs, such as Cytoxan® (cyclophosphamide), methotrexate, Cladribine® (leustatin), and Imuran® (azathioprine). These agents have a long history of success in other autoimmune diseases like lupus and rheumatoid arthritis.

If the ABC + R drugs alone don't seem to be stopping relapses and if they are becoming progressively more severe and debilitating—it may be the right time to think "combo." A good MS specialist will know when to try a combo and when to leave things alone. Both of you need to be informed. Both of you need to discuss the different treatment plans. Both of you should know your options and the pros and cons of each.

But medicine alone will not keep multiple sclerosis symptoms at bay. Rehabilitation can help you function at a higher level—and offer you a better quality of life. It's time to discover "the other half" of multiple sclerosis treatment.

CHAPTER NINE

WHY REHABILITATION?

*I thought I'd get along just fine with my new drug
and regular checkups. But I really hated the way I
walked. I was wobbly and I had no strength. And I
was really tired all the time. I couldn't get any work
done! I'm glad my doctor recommended a rehabilitation center that specialized in MS. I go there as an
outpatient a few days a week and I have to say,
within weeks, I was walking better—and I had
learned some good strategies to keep fatigue from
winning. I can't believe how important rehabilitation
turned out to be! Now I really feel like I'm in
control—and not my disease.*

—A 32-year-old female lawyer who came
to learn the benefits of rehabilitation

• *Fact:* In 1999, a study by Dr. A. Solari in Milan, Italy,
published in *Neurology*, found that there was a significant improvement in people with MS who get rehabilitation. Fifty MS patients who could walk, but not well,
were divided into two groups; each had not had one or
more episodes (relapses) within the prior three months
nor had they been treated with immunotherapy drugs in
the past six months. None of them had significant cognitive impairment. One group was given exercise programs to use at home. The other group was admitted to
a rehabilitation hospital. *At the end of three weeks, the
group that had been treated with a formal rehabilitation program had significantly increased their FIM
motor score (a measure of functional independence)*

and decreased their overall disability. Their quality of life and self-esteem had also increased.

- *Fact:* A study done by Dr. J. Freeman and his colleagues at the Institute of Neurology in London and published in *Neurology* in 1999 found even better results. They studied 50 patients with progressive MS who had just been discharged from inpatient rehabilitation. Using a battery of tests that measured neurological status, disability, quality of life, and emotional well-being, Dr. Freeman and his colleagues discovered that *one year after their rehabilitation—and despite relapses that left them more impaired—the patients' emotional well-being and quality of life continued to be maintained for seven to ten months after discharge.* The people in the study also made significant gains in their general health.

- *Fact:* In another study done by Dr. Freeman and his colleagues published in the *Annals of Neurology* in 1997, 66 people with secondary-progressive MS were either admitted to a rehabilitation center for 25 days or they were put on a waiting list and didn't get to go. After six weeks, even though the level of impairment was the same for all 66 people tested, *the people who had 25 days of rehabilitation significantly increased their level of disability and handicap—and increased their functional status as well.*

- *Fact:* A study published in *Multiple Sclerosis* in April 1999 found that *those people with secondary and primary progressive MS who had formal rehabilitation improved their cognitive functions by 57%.*

And there's more. . . . Study after study shows that rehabilitation can improve the quality of life of a person with MS.

From the ability to perform the activities of daily living to a sense of well-being, from mobility to cognitive skills—rehabilitation, combined with disease-modifying medication, can make all the difference in the life of a person with multiple sclerosis. Rehabilitation can make life easier.

REHABILITATION THAT WORKS

It's true that once an axon is severed or severely damaged, it cannot spring back to life. An impairment caused by a multiple sclerosis attack does not always disappear once the episode is over. There may be residual impairment; impairments sometimes become worse.

Rehabilitation provides the skills, the strategies, and the exercises you need to lessen the impact of your impairments on your life. Rehabilitation helps you with physical, emotional, and cognitive problems—as well as with the problems that most affect our self-esteem: bladder and bowel problems, sexual dysfunction, and the performance of such simple tasks as eating, taking a shower, and getting dressed.

In short, rehabilitation helps give you back some of what you have lost. New ways to do old tasks. New ways to cope and move forward.

REHABILITATION FOR MS: A SLIGHTLY DIFFERENT COURSE

Rehabilitation has been proven to help any person who has become incapacitated. Whether it be a traumatic injury to someone's brain or spinal cord or a sudden stroke—a period of time in a good rehabilitation facility can teach everything from new cognitive skills to finding a new career. But multiple sclerosis is slightly different. A person with MS has a variety of problems—none of which can be handled in a 15-minute visit with the neurologist.

HOW DO YOU CHOOSE A GOOD NEUROLOGIST?

The neurologist is your first line of defense—and the one you choose can make all the difference between controlling your disease and becoming a victim. Look for these qualities when you go "shopping":

- Knowledgeable and passionate *about MS*
- Aggressive and ready to intervene *immediately*
- Ready to answer all your questions *without looking at her watch*
- Prepared to refer you *to a good therapist or specialist for a specific problem*
- Involved *in the community*
- Associated with *a hospital, clinic, or rehabilitation center*
- A person you respect, admire *and with whom you feel comfortable*
- Board certified *or board eligible: The National Multiple Sclerosis Society has a formal process for including neurologists on their referral list. Call 1-800-FIGHT-MS and press or say one (1) to reach your local chapter and find out more.*

The level of disability varies from person to person; there can be psychological issues, physical problems, or environmental difficulties. MS is not just weakness or the loss of vision. The disease must be seen in the context of who you are, what your personality is like, how you can best handle your disability—while offering the best information on support groups, financial burdens, and cutting-edge therapies.

Perhaps your first episode is mild, with symptoms that require care from knowledgeable therapists—but not an overnight stay. An outpatient Multiple Sclerosis Center can be ideal in a situation like this: Supervised by a neurologist, you are able to get all the appropriate medical treatments, including disease-modifying drugs. In addition, you also get the expertise of a rehabilitation staff—who can provide testing, evaluation, and education for your condition; counseling for depression; physical therapy to help with any residual tremors or balance problems; advice and advocacy for dealing with the health insurance bureaucracy; insight on community support; even strategies to keep exercise from fatiguing you or making you feel uncomfortably hot. All this under one roof!

Outpatient rehabilitation can be done once a week, three times a week (as much as up to five days a week) for a few hours, half a day, or even a full day—whatever is required for you to increase your quality of life and your knowledge base.

The staff of an MS center is always there for you, for follow-up interviews and evaluations, as well as for possible future episodes. They recognize you as an individual—and treat your disease as such. And, if need be, the center also has inpatient rehabilitation facilities, where the different areas of rehabilitation are intensified and you can learn new skills and adaptive strategies for your MS. Inpatient rehabilitation can offer continuous therapy for spasticity, speech problems, cognitive dysfunction, bladder and bowel problems, severe fatigue—even in-depth exercises and information for using the right wheelchair.

REHAB STEP-BY-STEP:
INTERVENTION AT VARIOUS STAGES OF MS

If you have been newly diagnosed with MS and the disease has a minimal impact on your life, you won't need the kind of rehabilitation someone whose MS has progressed to the point where it is interfering with the quality of life. Here are the three different types of intervention a good rehabiliation team will do:

1. *Newly Diagnosed/Minimal Impact:* This type of rehab will concentrate on the physical—maximizing your strength and making you more fit. The team will develop an exercise program specifically designed to offset your MS symptoms and prevent you from overexerting yourself—while still doing your personal best. You may also work with a neuropsychologist, so as to establish a baseline of your cognitive abilities. He or someone on his team will help you adjust to your new disease and assist you with developing proper strategies to cope with the new stressors in your life. The team will also use this time to help you think about the future—and the activities of daily life that may be affected. They may help you decide to opt for an apartment on a ground floor, for example, or to take a job that doesn't require you to be on your feet all day long. You'll be given information on community resources and insurance polices—as well as the treatment options available to you.

2. *Moderate Impact:* Relapsing/remitting MS requires more of the same—plus added exercises to provide strength and endurance. Your rehabilitation team will

be able to offer you with the focus and resources you need—working as one, working as a smooth-running team. Your neuropsychological support will continue to see if your symptoms have gotten worse—and if cognitive rehabilitation is required. You will learn how to manage not only your physical and cognitive symptoms—but also how to compensate for your disability in all the activities of daily life: driving, personal hygiene, work, leisure time, and home life. *(See Chapter 14 for information on these ADLs—activities of daily living—and adaptive equipment).*

3. ***Advanced Progression:*** There is no question that a good rehabilitation center is necessary if your MS has progressed to the point where your disabilities are pronounced. At this point, your team will help devise range-of-motion exercises and help you learn proper positioning in your scooter or wheelchair. You will have your nutrition analyzed and adjusted; you will learn what equipment you need—and how to use it at home and at work. You and your family will also receive information and advice on everything from safety issues to correct transferring from wheelchair to bed training, from proper skin care to bladder and bowel management, from coping with spasticity to dealing with mobility issues.

THE CLUES TO A GOOD REHABILITATION CENTER

There are six "golden" goals that every good MS Rehabilitation Center and every good therapist on staff must strive to achieve:

Golden Goal #1: Improve Fitness and Condition

Imagine if you were a person with secondary-progressive MS—and you were made stronger by improving your endurance! What an amazing feeling of control—and a very real measurement of improved function.

Golden Goal #2: Improve Activities of Daily Living (ADLs)

These are the foundations of reclaiming your self-esteem: Going to the bathroom. Dressing yourself. Preparing food. Taking a shower. Cleaning a room. Managing a checkbook. Buying groceries and more.

HELP! THERE'S NO MS CENTER NEAR ME

If you do not live near an MS center, you can work with your neurologist to get referrals for the right therapists and to make sure that their files and progress reports are given to your doctor. You can also work with a regular rehabilitation center; all of them are equipped to handle the impairments that can come from disease or trauma.

Your local chapter of the National Multiple Sclerosis Society can also help—providing recommendations, support groups within the community, community services, and up-to-the-minute educational materials. Call 1-800-FIGHT MS and press or say "one" to be directly connected to your local chapter.

Golden Goal #3: Reduce Anxiety and Depression

A disability can plunge you into despair: the fact that you cannot dress yourself or walk or be as independent as you once were can hurt. The disease itself can create anxiety: When will my next attack occur? Will it be worse than this one? A good rehabilitation facility will be able to provide therapy, medical treatment, and strategies to help you cope with these very real feelings.

Golden Goal #4: Provide a Sense of Well-Being

A sense of pride. Self-respect. Dignity. We all need these things. A good feeling is not as easily measured as a 25-foot walk, but it is just as important for maximum function. A first-class MS rehabilitation center is always thinking of building up your self-esteem as you do your exercises.

Golden Goal #5: Reduce Fatigue

As the number one symptom of MS, fatigue must be dealt with at a rehabilitation center. You will be provided with adaptive equipment, strategies, and suggestions for energy conservation, even medication, if necessary.

Golden Goal #6: Improve Overall Strength

Weakness is another common symptom of MS. Building up your strength will help in all other areas of your rehabilitation: growing self-esteem, reducing anxiety, and giving you a burst of energy. Remember: There are always reserves. People don't begin on empty—even when starting a rehabilitation program. A good rehab center will find that reserve and teach you how to use it!

A TEAM APPROACH

No one person could achieve all six goals by himself. Nor can rehabilitation take place in a vacuum. A rehabilitation center should and must have a variety of specialists who work with you and each other to maximize your abilities and the time you spend under their roof.

Rehabilitation is and must be a multidisciplinary program. A multidisciplinary approach not only reinforces vital skills, but keeps motivation strong as well. Depression, a very real symptom of MS, must be treated at the same time a patient's walking skills are worked on to keep the desire for progress strong.

The rehabilitation team works together, implementing and reinforcing an interrelated approach. The physical therapist knows the progress a patient is making with her slurred speech. The occupational therapist knows how she is handling her depression. The rehabilitation nurse knows the strategies that have been working to control her bladder. Each team member works in concert with the others, in communication with the others, even working side by side with the others. This makes sense: as a patient learns to use a scooter or a wheelchair, she might also be learning how to cope with her fatigue. As he learns to open a drawer with his weakened hands, he is also learning how to manage his constipation.

This multidisciplinary approach follows you through from the first day you enter the rehabilitation hospital to the day you become an outpatient—and beyond. Inpatient facilities work with outpatient facilities. And both work with the community at large—from your family and friends to your local chapter of the National Multiple Sclerosis Society. Dialogue is always open. As things change, you are not alone. Ever.

YOUR REHABILITATION TEAM PLAYERS

Now that you know the process of rehabilitation, you need to know who is doing it! As the saying goes, a team is only as good as its individual players. Let's take a quick look at the members of your rehabilitation team:

The neurologist or physiatrist. This is the leader, the physician who oversees it all: arranging medical tests, managing medication, deciding which clinical course of action is right for you, supervising the team. Ideally, your neurologist will specialize in multiple sclerosis and will be connected to a rehabilitation facility. While the neurologist manages your medication, he may also seek the consultation of a physiatrist, who specializes in physical medicine and rehabilitation. Sometimes two heads are better than one.

The rehabilitation nurse. In addition to tending to your medical needs, training you to use a disease-modifying drug injection, and helping you with bladder and bowel control, she will also be there to help, to listen, to inform when therapy is not in session. She can help reinforce your therapy goals: assisting you in transferring from a wheelchair to your bed, helping you eat with a knife and fork. Along with all the other team players, she will also help reduce your pain and reinforce pain management.

The physical therapist. This therapist does what it sounds like: treats and concentrates on physical movement. She will help an MS patient recover and maintain motor function; work on walking, balance and coordination; learn how to use a cane, scooter, or wheelchair; enhance strength, endurance, spasticity, and posture. She will also work out an exercise regimen for you, one that does not tire you out too much or create undue heat sensitivity. One of the most popular and safest forms of exercise for MS patients is aqua aerobics and strength–training *(which we'll be discussing in the next chapter)*.

The occupational therapist. This is the person most involved in your activities of daily living. She will help you learn how to use adaptive equipment and strategies to perform the simple routines of life at home: bladder and bowel function, personal hygiene, dressing, eating, swallowing, and, if possible, driving a car. She also provides exercises for finger and hand control, eye-hand coordination, energy management, and more. She will also teach you strategies to avoid falling and injuring yourself. In short, the occupational therapist teaches those functions that help a person with MS function in the community.

The neuropsychologist. This doctor studies the special relationship between the brain and behavior. She will perform neuropsychological diagnostic tests to evaluate your cognitive abilities, behavioral problems, and psychological structure. She and her staff will also provide individual, family, and group therapies specifically geared to people with disabilities.

The rehabilitation counselor. This person is a behavioral kingpin. He is very much involved in the emotional implications of your disease. Are you angry? Overly anxious? Lethargic and depressed? The rehabilitation counselor provides therapy that treats specific behavioral problems. A good counselor is also very much involved with the family.

He will work with them, offering strategies that help their loved one cope better—and help them cope better as well. He will help you and your loved ones understand the disease and what the future may hold.

The speech therapist. This therapist evaluates and treats all abilities pertaining to language: using it, comprehending it, reading it, writing it, and producing its sounds. He will help with slurred words and difficulties in forming words. He will also be heavily involved in the cognitive aspects of rehabilitation, determining if you have any cognitive impairments when it comes to memory, abstract reasoning, decision-making, attention span, even social interaction—all to better help you interact in a social setting once again. Speech therapists are also specialists in swallowing; they can also evaluate and treat any swallowing problem you may experience.

The vocational specialist. Independence is an important element in the rehabilitation credo, and this therapist helps a patient reach it. If your MS is progressive, he will help you reevaluate your goals and see how you can either adapt your limitations to your career, or transfer your skills to a different line of work. He can help you reenter the community in a more positive away. Frequently, this person comes to a rehabilitation center from an outside community agency.

The clinical dietitian. Proper nutrition is important for good health. If you have MS, it becomes even more important to live a healthy lifestyle, eating foods that provide proper nutrition, energy, and strength (and fiber for bowel problems!) The dietitian can also provide instructions for a special diet if you are having swallowing difficulties.

The respiratory therapist. This therapist provides care if you have difficulty breathing, to help ward off complications and infections such as pneumonia.

The case manager. Memorize the name. This is your medical and financial advocate. You and your family will be in close contact with this team member. This is the person you will turn to with questions, problems, and needs. The case manager is also your liaison between you and the rest of the staff, between you and your health insurance plan. A case manager will explain the different kinds of therapies to the entire family. She will provide the names and addresses of support groups. She will offer understanding and sensitivity. She will work with the financial issues. And, most important of all, the case manager will stick by you. In the future, between relapses, long after you are home, the case manager will be there if you have a question, a problem, or simply a need to talk.

HE SAYS IT ALL

Rehabilitation differs from many specialties in that it is an active process of education whereby the disabled persons acquire and use knowledge and skills to optimize their physical, psychological, and social function.

—Dr. J. A. Freeman

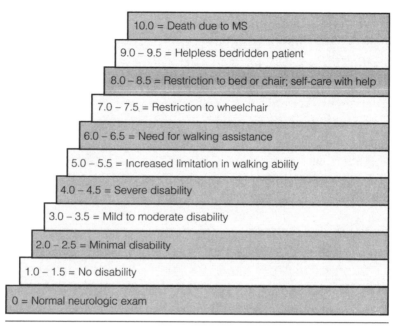

10.0 = Death due to MS

9.0 – 9.5 = Helpless bedridden patient

8.0 – 8.5 = Restriction to bed or chair; self-care with help

7.0 – 7.5 = Restriction to wheelchair

6.0 – 6.5 = Need for walking assistance

5.0 – 5.5 = Increased limitation in walking ability

4.0 – 4.5 = Severe disability

3.0 – 3.5 = Mild to moderate disability

2.0 – 2.5 = Minimal disability

1.0 – 1.5 = No disability

0 = Normal neurologic exam

Expanded Disability Status Scale

DETERMINING YOUR DISABILITY

In order to know where to start in your rehabilitation program, your team has to use some form of measurement. The one universally recognized by insurance companies and the Food and Drug Administration (to approve the results of clinical drug trials) is the Expanded Disability Status Scale (EDSS).

Although the EDSS Scale helps measure disability, it concentrates on mobility—not self-esteem or the activities of daily living. A better measurement used by rehabilitation centers to assess a person's improvement is the FIM—or

Functional **I**ndependence **M**easure. This evaluation pinpoints your ability to take care of yourself—and how well you can move around. The more impairment from your MS episode, the less independent you will be and the lower your FIM score. Your score will also show your improvement as you make functional gains; it can help your rehabilitation team determine if you are left with any residual impairments—and how much of each. FIM is a highly detailed assessment involving all rehabilitation disciplines. It uses 18 categories, including:

- Feeding yourself
- Bathing
- Personal grooming
- Dressing
- Controlling your bladder and bowel
- Problem solving
- Walking solo or with cane, scooter, or wheelchair assistance
- Ability to move from a chair to a bed
- Comprehension
- Expression

Each of these categories is given a score, on a 7-point scale that ranges from total assistance (1) to total independence (7). FIM can draw a fairly accurate picture of your functional abilities and track them through the entire rehabilitation process—and beyond.

FIM is one of the most current and most reliable of the functional tests. It is used in rehabilitation hospitals and clinics across the country. Many facilities also use a Quality of Life tool to measure how well you view your current situation—at work, at home, at play.

A SAMPLE PLAN FOR TREATMENT AND GOALS FOR AN MS PATIENT

This is a basic "checklist" our rehabilitation team players use when a person with MS comes to one of our HealthSouth rehabilitation facilities:

Daily Medical Supervision to:

- *Establish effective bowel and bladder management program*
- *Establish effective spasticity management program*
- *Establish effective pain management regime*

Daily Physical, Occupational, and Speech Therapy Program to:

- *Maintain/increase range-of-motion of all extremities*
- *Improve balance*
- *Increase strength of trunk and extremities*
- *Increase independence in ADLs*
- *Increase independence and safety in position changes and transfers*
- *Make a complete orthotic assessment*
- *Improve ambulation and gait pattern*
- *Increase endurance in wheelchair mobility*
- *Complete cognitive assessment and provide therapy as indicated*
- *Improve speech intelligibility*
- *Specify appropriate, durable medical equipment*
- *Provide patient/family/caretaker education*

You now know the score on rehabilitation. You can recognize a good rehabilitation center and you know how to choose a doctor. You know what to expect from a rehab facility and you know how much it can help. We'll now go over some of the more common problems people with MS encounter—and how a rehabilitation center can help.

CHAPTER TEN

MOBILITY IN MS: WALKING, SPASTICITY, WEAKNESS, TREMORS, AND MORE

*I just found something new—and I love it: water aer-
obics! When I'm in the water, I feel weightless. My
arms and legs are as graceful as a ballerina's. I have
no disability, nothing. I don't even get too tired or
hot. Another plus: It's good for my heart. I thank my
physical therapist every day!*

—A 51-year-old homemaker with
relapsing-remitting MS who goes to
a HealthSouth MS Center three times a week

John was fit as a fiddle. In fact, he took great pride in his
body: His arm muscles were developed and his stomach was
washboard-tight. He'd always had a good body because he'd
always been active. As a teenager, he was a star athlete; the
best runner on his track and field team. He was competitive.
He loved races—and he usually won.

When John wasn't racing, he could be found tinkering with
the family car or his brother's motorcycle (when his brother
wasn't looking!) It made sense that when John graduated
high school, he made his love for driving profitable by becoming a mechanic.

And he made his love of motorcycles a part of his life:
every weekend, he would ride his beloved Harley in any race
within a 300-mile radius of home.

John figured there was nothing missing in his life: He had
his cars, his motorcycle; and, most importantly, he even had

a great wife and a newborn baby. There was nothing more he wanted. He was content.

That's why he was so disconcerted when, just like that, his speech started to slur. His vision blurred, and he had trouble walking without holding on to something. What was going on here?

Since John had never been to a doctor in his life (except maybe when he was a baby and had no choice), he just ignored the symptoms. Figured it was the flu. Or maybe he had hurt his head racing the past weekend. Whatever it was, John chose to ignore it. It was nothing. He didn't even mention his symptoms to his wife.

John felt he must have been right because just as suddenly as the symptoms came, they went away. He was fine. Better than fine. . . .

At least for the next six months—when his symptoms flared up again. This time it was worse; he couldn't even walk to the car to go to work. He missed work for one of the first times in his life. Worse, that weekend he almost had a fatal crash on his motorcycle!

John's wife insisted: he had to see a doctor now. John didn't argue. Something was definitely going on and he was scared. . . .

His doctor referred him to a neurologist who had him take an MRI. Sure enough: The MRI showed multiple lesions in his brain. He needed to take some serious medicine now.

The neurologist started him on powerful steroids; they relieved the symptoms and he started to feel better. When the doctor suggested that John start one of the ABC + R disease-modifying drugs to help halt the frequency and seriousness of his attacks, John shook his head. Forget about it!

First of all, John got better all by himself last time. He didn't need to take any medicine then and he didn't have to now. The steroids were enough! Besides, he was embarrassed to tell his doctor that he was afraid of needles. There he was: this big star athlete with a needle phobia! No way could he give himself the injections the disease-modifying drugs required.

John went back to his life. He was better, but not 100%. His balance was a little off and his speech was a little slow. But all seemed well. . . .

Wham! Nine months later John was hit with a much worse MS attack. His legs became numb and so weak that he couldn't walk at all. He had difficulty holding objects and opening containers.

This time John's neurologist put him in the hospital and once again gave him IV steroid treatment. Unfortunately, this time his symptoms only slightly improved. John then did a few weeks of rehabilitation and it helped: He was better able to take care of himself. Thank goodness for rehab!

Perhaps if John had started disease-modifying therapy, this attack might have been less severe. Although there is no way to know for sure, the good news is that John has changed his behavior. He now goes to his rehabilitation center three times a week and hasn't missed a day yet. He is also taking his disease-modifying injections on a regular basis.

As this scenario shows: you can only sweep things under the rug for so long. Eventually, there's no more room. But it's not all doom and gloom for John—or for other people with MS who need help getting around.

You have already learned about the benefits of rehabilitation. Now we're going to get specific. This chapter is all about mobility and how an entire rehabilitation team works together to get you moving.

THE PHYSICAL THERAPY CREDO: SEM

No matter what the problem, no matter what the condition, no matter what or when physical therapy is required, the goal is always the same: physical independence. This is acquired through various therapies that work on what we call the SEM factor:

- *Strength.* One of the more common symptoms of MS is weakness. Your muscles need to be built up and toned—and your movements coordinated.
- *Endurance.* Another major symptom of MS is fatigue—which can lead to inactivity. While your occupational therapist is working on energy management with you, your physical therapist will be creating a specific exercise program designed to improve function—and keep you going for longer periods of time. The program will usually involve water exercise and stretching exercises to keep you flexible and increase your range-of-motion.
- *Mobility.* The major key to physical independence is being able to move around, to get from one place to another. A physical therapist will evaluate your capabilities and help you improve your gait. If necessary, she will also show you how to use adaptive equipment specific to your needs: a lightweight brace, a cane, or a scooter.

MS symptoms such as numbness or tingling, weakness or spasticity, fatigue or heat intolerance, and lack of coordination, tremors, or loss of balance (ataxia) can all hinder your ability to walk—or even get around.

Let's go over the mobility issues that may arise when you have MS—and how a rehabilitation team can help:

WEAK IN THE KNEES: WEAKNESS AS A SYMPTOM OF MS

Muscle weakness is a very real problem for people who have MS; it causes gait problems and it may be linked to spasticity, loss of balance, and fatigue. But before you plunge into an exercise regimen, it's important for your physical therapist—and the entire rehabilitation team—to determine which muscles are weak and what factors are contributing to your gait problems.

Fortunately, there are several things your physical therapist can do to help with your muscle weakness. She can create an exercise program, combining aerobics and weight-lifting (progressive resistive exercise), that stops you just short of fatigue. A crucial rule for people who have MS and begin an exercise program:

Lifting weights or performing aerobic-intensive exercise to the point of fatigue like you did in the past may not be the best strategy now. You may feel weaker or fatigued after performing these activities, taking longer for recovery of your baseline.

On the other hand, performing little or no exercise can result in disuse weakness or muscle atrophy—which can further limit your function.

Working with the other members of the rehabilitation team, your physical therapist will devise a program that's just right: It won't fatigue you too much, and it will give your muscles the exercise they need. *(See the next chapter for exercise and fatigue management.)*

IF THESE LEGS COULD WALK:
ATAXIA, WEAKNESS, AND LACK OF COORDINATION

The mind might be willing, but the legs might be shaky. You might feel unbalanced and weak. Or you might walk awkwardly with your feet farther apart to give your body more support. This walking impairment is called ataxia and, although it can't be cured, we have strategies to help compensate for your problems. This is also true if you have a "foot drop," a common impairment in which weakness in the lower leg muscles causes the toes to drag and makes tripping or falling more likely. Compensatory devices become imperative.

It's important not to think of these devices as a sign of failure, a "giving up and giving in" to your disease. Instead, think of them as tools. Carpenters have their tools. So do painters. Computer programmers. Housekeepers. In every case, the tools help make their job easier, more efficient, and faster.

It's exactly the same with mobility.

Some of the "tools of the trade" you might need include:

Essential Tool #1: Shoes
If you have any problems with walking, a good, proper shoe is essential. Therapists recommend either rubber or leather-soled oxfords. Laces give a nice stability to your feet, but if

your hands are weakened, you might want to use Velcro straps. Soles are either rubber or leather; your gait pattern may make leather slippery on a smooth surface or make rubber stick to carpeting. Your choice depends on your walking problem. Consult with your therapist and remember that function is more important than fashion. The good news— many companies now make shoes that are both functional and fashionable.

Essential Tool #2: Orthotics

In addition to your sturdy, comfortable shoe, you might need a brace to help you walk without losing your balance. A molded ankle-foot orthosis (AFO) travels up from the sole of the foot, behind the calf, to below the knee. It is made of plastic and usually is individually designed to fit inside your shoe. (You can purchase shoes one-half size larger to accommodate your AFO.) The AFO will help:

- Decrease spasticity *(see the next section)* by forcing your foot to tilt at a specific angle
- Keep your foot from turning in or out (inversion or eversion) for extra stability
- Ease your fatigue
- Provide support for weakened muscles
- Create a proper gait for you
- Correct posture

If your ankle is very stiff, you might need additional support from a metal brace that fits around the outside of your shoe. This brace (called a Klenzak brace) is "spring loaded" to keep your toe from dropping. Today, you can get the same effect with lighter materials, including plastic and aluminum.

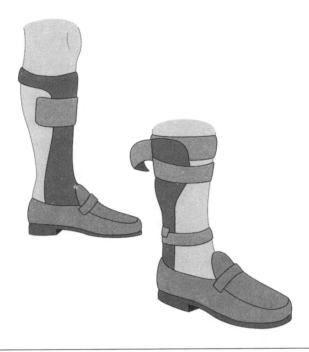

Rigid Polypropylene Ankle-Foot Orthosis

But what if your hip muscles are weak? Is it still possible to walk without feeling fatigued? Is it possible to walk at all? Yes! When you have a weakened hip, your gait will look as if you are doing a dance step: you will swing your leg out in front to allow your foot to touch the ground. To keep your balance, your knee might be forced back farther than it should, resulting in added stress (hyperextension) and, ultimately, painful joints. To avoid this condition you can use a Swedish hyperextension cage (a plastic form molded to your leg) to prevent you from snapping your knee back. If the knee cage doesn't work, all is not lost. A custom-made knee brace may do the job.

Essential Tool #3: Canes and Walkers

Braces and sturdy shoes can help keep fatigue at bay. They can also help you walk independently with a fairly stress-free gait. But if balance is also an issue, you might need a cane.

As your physical therapist will tell you, always hold your cane on your "good side." First advance the cane, then the affected leg, and finally, the unaffected leg.

WALKING AROUND: STAIRS, CURBS, AND GREEN, GREEN GRASS

When it comes to stairs, always think "Down with the bad, up with the good." When coming down the stairs, use your weak leg first, then your stronger one. If there's a railing, move your hand forward first, then step down. When going up, the stronger leg should go first.

Curbs are like stairs: "Down with the bad and up with the good."

Various surfaces can also present a challenge. Tile and linoleum are actually easier to walk on than carpeting. You should look down and make sure that a carpet is secured so it won't slide—and you won't fall. (As a matter of fact, get rid of all those loose throw rugs ASAP!)

Grass can feel strange at first, but knowing you're about to step on the green can take away the surprise element and you can keep your balance. Always lift your weak leg higher on difficult terrains.

And never go out alone if the surface is slippery! The number of people who come to a HealthSouth rehabilitation facility for a fractured hip after an ice storm is surprisingly high.

If you have weakness in both your legs, you might need to use two canes. (Remember, these are only tools. They are designed to make you less weak and less tired.) The left foot and right hand move forward together; the right foot and left hand move work together. If your balance and weakness are more severe, you may need to use Lofstrand crutches. These forearm crutches offer more stability than a plain cane; they also won't weaken your upper body as much. Again, left and right go together.

Walkers can be a boon if your balance is bad. Walk forward with arms extended, first the weak leg, then the strong one. If your gait is particularly off, you should stay away from walkers with wheels. We have found that putting old tennis balls over the rear wheels of a walker allows the walker to "glide" more slowly and not get away from you.

Essential Tool #4: Scooters and Wheelchairs

Scooters are one of the best inventions ever made for people with MS. They don't have the stigma that wheelchairs are perceived to have. Practical and easy-to-use, motorized scooters also keep you from getting fatigued, and they don't require a lot of hand-leg coordination. But scooters are only good for people who may have difficulty walking, but can still get around their houses or apartments. Scooters aren't designed for sitting in all day long.

If you can't walk at all and need assistance supporting your body, you can still find mobility and independence in a motorized wheelchair. Although a scooter may look more fashionable, you will be more comfortable with all the right seating options that a wheelchair provides.

Your physical therapist will help you choose the right mode of transportation; he will also give you "driving

WINNEY, NOT POOH

A "winney" is not just a character in a children's story. In fact it can be downright practical. A case in point: the Winney walker. This apparatus can double as a walker with brakes and as a "grocery cart" you can wheel around and use to hold packages. But don't use one if you have balance problems; it won't offer enough support.

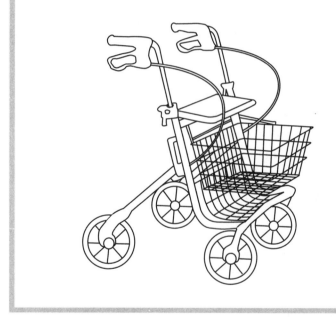

lessons." These are the elements to look for when picking out a good scooter or wheelchair:

- *Control.* You have to feel secure in your wheelchair or scooter—and this means it must provide the right amount of control you need for your specific mobility concerns. Perhaps you need speed to move around your office or to cross the street. Or maybe your house has a lot of twists and turns. Or maybe you live in an apartment house with long, wide hallways. Whatever the scenario, you'll need a mode of transportation that helps you change direction smoothly—and helps you stay in charge. Think of it as a vehicle to take you where you want to go as easily and efficiently as possible.

- *Tires.* Obviously, tires are a vital element in any working wheelchair or scooter. You need wheels that move smoothly—and that means good, durable tires. In the same way you'd choose tires for your new car, you want the best for your new vehicle: a tire that holds up, that won't easily puncture or lose air, that has enough tread for the terrains you use: pavement, snow, sand, cobblestones, or gravel.

- *Brakes.* As much as you want to move, you also want to stop whenever you want. You don't want your scooter or your wheelchair to roll when you transfer to a bed or chair. As with your car, your scooter or wheelchair brakes are vital for your safety. And, as with your car, they must be adjusted and tested periodically. Make sure you are able to use your breaks easily to stop your wheels, and that it isn't too difficult to engage them. Scooters have hand brakes similar to those on a bicycle. (Make sure they aren't too tight: you don't want to get fatigued.)

- *Leg Rests and Foot Rests.* If you are in your wheelchair or scooter for a good portion of the day, it becomes imperative that your feet are comfortably placed at an angle that keeps your circulation going, prevents pressure sores, and reduces any spasticity or swelling. Your footrests should be aligned so that your knees are slightly higher than your hips. This is the optimum position for balance and for keeping fatigue at bay. The main types of leg rests and foot rests are:

√ *Wheelchair swing-away foot rests and leg rests.* These are exactly as they sound. To disengage, the left and right rests "swing away" from each other; this makes transfers or standing easier.

√ *Wheelchair elevating leg rests.* These adjustable items allow you to move your legs further away from the chair, closer to you, or higher and lower. They are especially good if you have swelling in your legs or feet.

√ *Wheelchair rigid adjustable footrests.* Rather than swinging away from each other, these foot rests are attached; you move them up or down for comfort. They are lightweight, efficient, and help you move quickly.

√ *Scooter foot rests.* Since your steering wheel is positioned between your legs (from the tiller wheel to your feet), you need foot rests that won't hit the wheel and that keep your knees and legs in a comfortable sitting position. Knees should be bent at the same level as the cushion.

• *Arm Rests.* Like your legs, your arms need a place to "sit" comfortably. This is especially important to prevent fatigue for already weakened arms. Look for adjustable-height armrests that can be positioned for your exact requirements. For scooters, this is

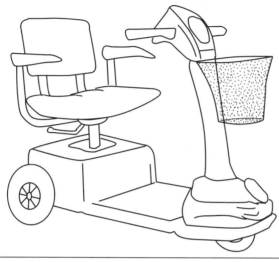

Electric Scooter

particularly important: Your arms must be positioned comfortably for your hands to hold the tiller-wheel bars—where your brakes are! They also need to swing away to make transferring easier.

- **Seats and Cushions.** You might already have the color and the fabric picked out, but unless your seat is comfortable, the most spectacular combo won't mean a thing. If you use your wheelchair or scooter a great deal during the day, it's crucial that your vehicle's seat does all the right things: keep pressure sores at bay, align your body, provide balance, offer efficient energy, decrease fatigue, and make you feel at ease. What to look for:

  √ *Seat Position.* Ideally you should be able to sit in your chair or scooter with your back to the frame and your knees bent; your knees should be slightly higher than your hips to help provide trunk control. This position provides easier reaching, propelling, and turning.

√ *Seat Cushion.* This should never be wider than the chair frame. Your legs should fit comfortably along the bottom of the seat frame, with your feet solidly positioned on their footrests. (The footrests will be smaller than your feet.) There are three main types of seat cushions:

1. *Roho,* which is an air-inflated rubber cushion that provides the best protection against skin irritations.
2. *Gel,* which is filled with gelatinous material that provides good support and body balance.
3. *Foam,* which is the most versatile: It can be shaped to your body and it's very light. (It's also the least expensive.)

√ *Seat covers are optional,* but they do protect your seat from the elements. They can also make an individual "fashion" statement when covered in your favorite fabric. Just be sure that the material is not abrasive or too easily bunched up; these types of fabrics can irritate your skin.

√ *Scooter Savvy.* Your legs should rest far enough away from the tiller wheel so it won't rub or irritate them.

• ***Pockets and Baskets.*** For extra convenience when shopping or doing errands, a basket in the back of your scooter or a pouch attached to the side of your wheelchair can be very helpful. You can also decorate and design them any way you want.

SPASTICITY TALKS

The weakened muscles, tremors, and loss of balance that can be part of MS are disabling enough. Add spasticity, an imbalance of muscle tension perceived as "stiffness", and it can be very difficult to get comfortable—let alone walk.

Almost all of us have seen people with spasticity. We can see the extra effort as they try to put one foot in front of another, as they try to move an arm or hand. It is as if their bodies have a mind of their own, forcing arms and legs to resist where their owners would like them to go.

Spasticity's imbalance of muscle tension affects our ability to move a muscle or group of muscles. For example, if a person with spasticity tries to straighten her elbow to put on her blouse, the muscles on one side of the elbow resist the movement, keeping the arm from moving in the desired direction. The result is a prolonged contraction, a tightness that can be extremely frustrating, and painful as well. Spasticity can make an arm or leg appear frozen in one position, hiding any underlying potential for movement.

Spasticity is increased by, and can cause, anxiety, a full bladder, urinary tract infections, pain, and constipation—all fairly common symptoms of multiple sclerosis. Your personal hygiene can be affected as you try to wash a clenched fist or tightly bent leg.

Worse, spasticity forces you to increase your energy expenditure. As you try to move that "frozen" leg or arm, you are using more energy than your body can handle, leading to fatigue. Medication can usually help, but there are other strategies that are useful as well.

SOUNDS LIKE . . .

It's not a contraction. It's a contracture—a painful muscular condition resulting from muscle weakness combined with a lack of movement. This combination causes the muscles and tendons to shorten and decrease their range of motion. When you have a contracture, it means that the muscles in your legs, ankles, or feet are shortened. This can cause even more mobility problems—and pain. The good news that orthotic devices, range-of-motion exercises, and anti-spasticity medicine can all help. In certain situations, surgery may be indicated.

Spasticity can be improved by range-of-motion exercises that concentrate on relaxing and loosening the tight, spastic muscles. These exercises are designed to:

- Decrease muscle tone—to improve muscle function
- Produce proper body position—to protect limbs from injury
- Prevent contractures
- Teach people with MS how to work with their spasticity, learning, for example, how to move or stand on a spastic leg. (This prevents the loss of too much tone—which can make the leg less useful.)

Other important treatments to help people with spasticity are (botulinum toxin) Botox® and intrathecal baclofen (ITB). Unfortunately, these are both under-utilized because many neurologists—and their MS patients—are either not fully aware of their value or simply don't think to use them. Instead, physicians may rely entirely on baclofen (Lioreseal®), tizanidine (Zanaflex®), sodium dantrolene (Dantrium®), clonazepam (Klonopin®), or cyclobenzaprine (Flexeril®). Although these medicines are very useful, they are not universally effective and may have side effects that include weakness and fatigue. Doctors should consider Botox® and ITB—for the right patient in the right situation.

BOTOX®: AN OLD FOE AND A NEW FRIEND

Although derived from the same toxin that could invade grandma's canned tomatoes, this highly diluted toxin can be safely injected into individual muscles of the arms and legs—weakening overactive muscles and allowing spastic, clenched fingers to open and tight, stiff legs to relax.

Botox® was first used to help people with ble-pharospasm (a condition involving overactive eyelids and frequent blinking). A few injections into the muscles of the eyelids and the blinking and eyelid over-activity could be controlled for at least three months at a time. It took only a small leap for physicians to realize that Botox® could be used to weaken other over-active muscles in other parts of the body. Think of it: your clenched fist, unable to fit through the sleeve of your blouse, may glide through more easily. . . . Or you can bend your leg more easily to put on your pants and shoes.

In short, Botox® can relax spastic muscles and decrease related pain. These more relaxed muscles, in turn, will allow you to do strengthening exercises to help counteract the weakness caused by MS. And, most important, although

Botox® may not necessarily return full function, *it can increase the quality of your life.*

Even the procedure itself is quite simple; it can be done on an outpatient basis. Using a very small, fine needle, your doctor pinpoints the overactive muscles and injects a small quantity of the clear liquid Botox®. The toxin moves a short distance and finds the place where the nerve enters the muscle and causes temporary weakness. It usually takes two to three weeks to first see any benefit and the resulting weakness is temporary—lasting only three to five months. Although this might not sound like good news, it very much is. Why? Because during this "weak" time, your physical therapist can work on exercises to keep your muscles loose and more functional—building up strength in your arm every day. Even if your spasticity proves to be stubborn, there's no reason to despair: Repeat injections can be performed as frequently as every three months There are no serious side effects from Botox®, and almost all insurance companies cover its use for these purposes.

Botox® works best in the smaller muscles of the arms because only limited amounts can be injected at one time. The larger muscles of the legs need a much greater amount of toxin—which is where intrathecal baclofen (ITB) comes into play.

ITB: SPASTICITY'S OTHER BEST FRIEND

ITB works best for spasticity in the lower extremities, the "antigravity" muscle groups: Calves, thighs, and buttocks—which is where people with MS are usually most affected. But many people with multiple sclerosis, especially those with secondary-progressive MS, may need both Botox® and ITB therapy: Botox® for the small muscles of the arms and hands and ITB for their legs. A perfect fit!

When taken orally, baclofen is a medicine that, in high doses, can cause weakness, dizziness, and drowsiness. In addition, baclofen is not as effective in brain spasticity as in spinal spasticity—and an MS patient may have both.

A small titanium pump, designed and produced by the Medtronic Corporation, overcomes these problems by directly placing tiny amounts of baclofen directly in the cerebrospinal fluid. The pump is about the size of a hockey puck and fits comfortably under the skin. The rate at which it delivers the baclofen can be adjusted as often as necessary by a doctor or nurse using a computer and circular wand that are placed over the skin. For some patients this procedure can produce a dramatic reduction in spasticity and pain.

To find out if you will benefit from ITB, your doctor may recommend a baclofen trial, which is done on an outpatient basis. A simple spinal tap is performed, which allows a small amount of baclofen to be inserted into your spinal fluid. Over the next few hours, a nurse and physical therapist will monitor you for any changes in your muscle tone. Change is good—even the slightest bit; the amount of change isn't as important as the fact that you get some response. If your spasticity decreases after the injection (as measured by a system called the Ashworth scale), you may be a candidate for implantation of an ITB pump.

ITB therapy has made a dramatic difference for many people with MS—decreasing the overactive tone in their legs and, ultimately, allowing them to walk, better transfer from wheelchair to bed to chair, sit properly in their scooter or wheelchair, and, most importantly, be free of pain.

The pump and its battery last five to seven years and are easily replaced in an outpatient procedure. The average person will return to the outpatient clinic every two to three months to have the pump refilled with baclofen—which involves tapping into the pump's reservoir via a simple injection, removing any remaining medicine, and refilling your "tank" for another two to three months of travel down the road. Since MS is characterized by relapses and remissions, your pump may need to be adjusted more frequently to fine tune your spasticity. Don't wait for your routine appointment: Go in earlier if you note changes that last more than a few days!

Although expensive, ITB therapy is generally covered by insurance. It can truly make a difference in your functional abilities—and your quality of life.

TREMORS

Yes, it was the name of a successful science fiction movie. But when your hands or feet are trembling, it's no fantasy. It's a disabling, inconvenient, and sometimes embarrassing reality.

Parkinson's disease is usually associated with tremors— the uncontrollable shaking of the head, a hand, or a foot. But tremors are also a common symptom of multiple sclerosis, one that can affect your hand coordination, mobility, and quality of life.

An MS tremor is different, however, from the more common Parkinsonian tremor. Instead of the uncontrollable trembling that occurs while you are at rest, either sitting or standing, which is common in Parkinson's Disease, an MS tremor is an intention tremor: It becomes active when you exert yourself. Lifting a cup of coffee to your mouth. Picking up a pen. Reaching out to shake a hand. Suddenly, as you perform these simple activities, you start to tremble. You also find yourself reaching past the point where you wanted to go. As you lift the coffee cup, the tremors cause you to miss your mouth, spilling the coffee on your lap. As you pick up the pen, you grab slightly further than you meant to; the pen seems impossible to pick up.

Tremors in people with MS are associated with lesions in the cerebellum of the brain—which also may cause a lack of coordination and imbalance.

YOUR TURN TO SPEAK

Sometimes tremors are less visible. Your lips, tongue, or jaw can also get tremors—which can affect your ability to speak. Tremors can interfere with your breath control, which, in turn, results in irregular speech. They can also impair your ability to speak above a whisper.

A speech therapist can help with voice and mouth exercises that increase your ability to communicate. She might have you read or sing out loud to help you modulate your words; she will help you control your breath; she will give you exercises that concentrate on your voice volume and pitch.

A device some speech therapists use is a paceboard—which literally is what it sounds like. A paceboard is a series of rectangles set next to each other; as you pronounce a syllable, you point to the paceboard. This will slow your speech and make it intelligible to others.

If you have tremors, your physical therapist may design balance exercises for you which will lessen the "shakes." Light weights that attach around your wrists with Velcro can also help. They add a sturdiness that may decrease the problem. On your ankles, weights may increase stability.

Weights, however, are controversial: Some physical therapists think they help the problem; others think they make things worse. The best solution? Try using weights for a few weeks and see if you improve. If so, continue on! If not, stop using them and concentrate instead on your balance exercises.

Medications can also help control tremors. Studies have found that certain anticonvulsants and antianxiety medications are the most effective. Unfortunately, they can cause sedation, depression, or affect cognition. Tell your doctor if you experience any side effects from your tremor medications. The ones prescribed most are: Klonopin®, Inderal®, Topamax®, BuSpar®, Mysoline®, and Atarax®.

TURNING THE HEAT UP

There is a common symptom of MS that can affect your ability to move: heat intolerance, or thermosensitivity. The amount of heat a person with MS can handle varies widely from individual to individual, but basically, thermosensitivity is the appearance of weakness or worsening symptoms as the body's core temperature rises. This can occur after just a short exposure to the heat of an August day, a hot bath, or even by exercise—which raises body temperature.

People who do not have MS sweat when they feel heat; they might pull off their sweatshirts as they continue to do their cardiovascular moves. But they can continue.

If you have MS, this elevation is not elation. Instead, it blocks the number of conducting fibers in your nervous system. You get hotter and hotter and feel more and more exhausted. The exact temperature at which this blocking occurs and the degree of impact on function varies from person to person.

You do not need to be walking on a treadmill to feel thermosensitivity. You can get the same results on hot, humid days and in tropical climates with minimal exertion

Although heat intolerance stops about one hour after you've exercised in most cases, the fatigue can last all day. *(See the next chapter for a detailed description of fatigue.)* And if your heat intolerance lasts longer than the amount of time you've exercised, you're doing too much!

The good news is that there are things, certain "cooling downs" that you can do to prevent heat intolerance from building up:

Cooling down #1: Pacing

We all know about pacing; it's what runners do when they run a marathon. It's what students should do when studying for finals. It's what people do to organize and pack for a trip. In other words, pacing is the way to plan your day. It involves realistic goals and plenty of rest periods. If you plan a realistic day, you'll be less likely to be left out in the heat.

Cooling down #2: Change Your Exercise Regimen

Instead of exercising two hours a day—which will ensure you "hit your heat intolerance wall," try exercising for only 30 minutes. But do that 30 minutes of exercise more frequently. In other words, 30 minutes five times a week will serve you better than two hours three times a week. (If that is too much, try 10 to 15 minutes at a time. Studies show this can work just as effectively as a workout in the gym!)

Cooling Down #3: Cooling Down Techniques

Instead of racing to the steam room, try a cool bath or shower after you've exercised. In fact, take that cool bath or shower before you begin your regimen to help keep heat intolerance at bay.

And be "weather smart": Avoid exercising outdoors in the middle of the day, especially if you live in a hot, humid climate.

Cooling Down #4: Use Adaptive Devices

There is a vast world of adaptive equipment out there to help you in your activities of daily living. *(See the next section for*

EXERCISE TIPS FOR PEOPLE WITH MS

Basically, the rules of common sense apply to everyone. But, if you have MS, you need to take a few precautions:

- *Wear loose-fitting, lightweight clothes. Avoid sweat suits—they'll only increase your heat overload.*
- *Exercise in cool temperatures. Water should be warm—not hot. Exercise rooms should have air conditioning.*
- *Take frequent breaks.*
- *Do chair or mat exercises if you are having difficulty with your balance. (Your physical therapist will help you modify your routines.)*
- *STOP if your MS symptoms start getting worse! And if you don't recover from these exercise side-effects, make sure you get a medical okay before starting up again.*

all the details.) Some of this equipment is designed specifically for heat intolerance, such as a cooling vest that you can
wear indoors or outdoors. Check out www.mscooling.org for
other items.

Cooling Down #5: Swim, Swim, Swim!

The best exercise for people with MS is water aerobics, water
fitness, water anything! Swimming in water at a temperature
of 86° F or less is well tolerated by most MS patients; some
people can tolerate even warmer water. You will have to
experiment to see what works best for you. Swimming is also
a great way to get into shape, helping your muscles get toned
and your heart pumping.

Cooling Down #6: Rate Your Perceived Exertion

One of the ways to make sure your workout is a good one—
not too strenuous to cause heat intolerance and not too easy
to forfeit any cardiovascular benefit—is to use your rate of
perceived exertion (RPE). It helps measure the intensity of
your workout so you can make changes if any symptoms
crop up. And best of all, *you* are in control of your workout
the whole time!

Basically, the RPE uses a range of 1 to 10, with 1 being very
light and 10 being to the max. While you are exercising, make
a mental note every so often as to where you are. Do you feel
as if your workout is too light? Are you exerting yourself too
much? Or does it feel just right, smack in the middle or a tad
higher.

Level	Definition
0	None
1	Very light
2	Light
3	Moderate
4	Somewhat heavy
5/6	Heavy
7/8	Very heavy
9	Extremely heavy
10	Maximum

Relative Perceived Exertion (RPE) Scale

WORKING OUT THE WORKOUT

To determine how much impairment you have—as well as to help design a personal exercise program for you—a physical therapist will evaluate your:

- *Coordination:* Do your hands and feet move easily as you walk?
- *Activity level:* Do you exercise regularly? Are you fit?
- *Muscle tone:* Are you strong? Have you ever lifted weights?
- *Balance and trunk stability:* Can you stand tall? Do you have proper posture and good sitting balance?

In creating an exercise regimen that's right for you, your physical therapist will work with the entire rehabilitation team to devise something that fits your MS progression. *(See Chapter 9 for more details.)* If your MS is newly diagnosed and has only a minimal impact on your life, your therapist

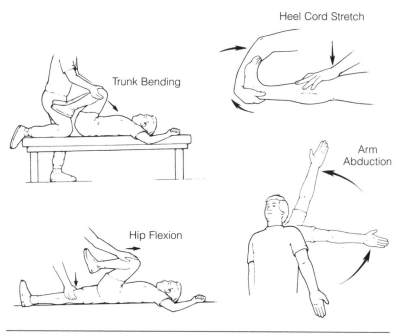

Range-of-Motion Exercises

will create a program that maximizes your strength and ensures that you are—and remain—physically fit. If your MS has progressed and has begun to have a moderate impact on your life, your therapist will concentrate on exercises that promote endurance and symptom management. If your MS has reached an advanced stage, your physical therapist will work on range-of-motion exercises; she will help you learn to transfer from wheelchair to bed; she will teach you proper positioning in your chair—as well as help the occupational therapist with any spasticity issues.

No matter what stage your MS is at, your physical therapist will use certain tools to keep you strong and build up your endurance. Some of these apparatus include parallel bars to help improve your gait, a big plastic Swiss ball to help strengthen your trunk and help regain posture realignment, water routines, range-of-motion stretching exercises, adjustable treadmills, and balance activities.

You now have a good idea of the symptoms that can cause mobility problems—and how they can be helped with rehabilitation. It's time now to check out another big symptom for people with MS, one that can affect your mobility and its success—as well as all your other rehabilitation goals. It's called fatigue.

CHAPTER ELEVEN

FATIGUE: WHY YOU FEEL TIRED AND WHAT YOU CAN DO ABOUT IT

*I find that I'm exhausted almost all the time. By late
afternoon I can barely keep my head up. It's hard to
figure out why: Is it the fact that I'm getting up there
in years–or is it my MS? And is it a symptom of my
MS—or a result of other symptoms?
Help! Whichever it is, I'm glad my rehabilitation
team has some time-tested solutions.*

—A 58-year-old firefighter with MS who is getting
treated for her fatigue at a HealthSouth facility.

Multiple sclerosis was an old friend to Elizabeth. She'd lived
with her disease for more than twenty years. And, at 56, she
now knew all the ins and outs of her condition. She knew the
signs and symptoms and how to decrease the intensity of her
attacks.

After all these years, Elizabeth had learned how to accept
her condition. When the fatigue caused by her MS became so
severe that she couldn't work a full day, she'd even gracefully
retired early from her high school history teacher position.

Three years ago, her physical therapist introduced her to
the scooter. She has been traveling around with it almost continuously now—but even her motorized method of independent travel didn't help her fatigue. She was exhausted all the
time.

When Elizabeth had first been diagnosed with MS, there
was little she could do about it. Disease-modifying drugs had

not yet been created and the only treatment available was steroids—and then only when she had an attack.

Unfortunately, because there was no medicine to help change the course of her MS, Elizabeth's relapses were no longer episodic; she now had secondary-progressive MS with little respite from her symptoms. When the ABC+R drugs came out, Elizabeth's neurologist immediately put her on a combination drug treatment (a chemotherapy drug and a disease-modifying medicine).

This new treatment might very well have slowed down her progression, but it was hard to tell. She was still so tired all the time! She couldn't do any housework for more than a half hour at a time. She couldn't do errands or go food shopping without frequent breaks. She couldn't even talk to her friends or watch TV without falling asleep!

Elizabeth was so frustrated by her constant fatigue that she became depressed; she lost weight and had trouble sleeping at night. Her neurologist added an antidepressant to her litany of drugs, but that was about all he could do to help.

Things changed when Elizabeth called the local chapter of the National Multiple Sclerosis Society. She discovered that there was a comprehensive MS Rehabilitation Center only five miles from her house. At last some hope!

Elizabeth got a referral and was soon introduced to a world where people truly understood her disease—and her constant fatigue. On her very first visit to the MS Center, she received a complete evaluation from a multi-disciplinary team of specialists and therapists. They were able to address not only her physical symptoms—but her social and psychological needs as well.

Today, Elizabeth still revs up her scooter and rides around town. But there is a crucial difference: energy. Thanks to the strategies she learned in rehabilitation, she has learned to preserve her energy. And her quality of life has vastly improved. She is living with her MS and managing it—rather than *it* managing her.

Elizabeth's situation is not unusual. Fatigue can rear its sleepy head in anyone who has MS—whether it be relapsing-remitting, secondary-progressive, or primary-progressive. Indeed, fatigue is so common a symptom that it isn't a stranger to anyone—those who have MS and those who don't.

But fatigue in MS is unique. Because of the MS lesions, nerves do not conduct electric impulses efficiently; nerve passageways become short-circuited. And this short-circuit can result in extreme fatigue. In fact, it can be so severe that a person with MS cannot even walk 100 yards without getting tired!

Nerve conduction is only part of the fatigue story. People with MS can also tire out from anxiety and stress to heat sensitivity, from difficulty in thinking to spastic, tense muscles. Their fatigue can even be a result of something we can all relate to: insomnia. In fact, the fatigue that comes with MS can have several different roots—all at the same time.

Let's go over the reasons for fatigue, the "Tiring Troubles" that affect so many people with MS—as well as the specific strategies you can use to conserve energy:

Tiring Trouble #1: "The Weakest Link" or Short Circuiting

When able-bodied people work out, they can experience weak muscles from too much weight training or from too many miles logged on the treadmill. This is a fact of life, one that is easily dealt with by staying away from exercise for a day or two, or cutting back on the intensity. People with MS, however, feel even more weakness in their limbs when they exercise—and even when they don't. That's because the nerves that control muscle and movement are "short-circuited." Their electrical impulses have been damaged thanks to multiple sclerosis lesions.

Energy Conservation Strategies: Aerobic exercises can help build endurance in your weakened muscles, but there is a fine line between "weak" and "strong." You need to plan your exercise time, provide plenty of rest, and only push yourself to the point before you start to fatigue. (If, for example, you find that your muscles buckle with weakness after 15 minutes on the Lifecycle®, go for only ten minutes instead.)

Tiring Trouble #2: "The Couch Potato Syndrome" or Deconditioning

There's an irony to muscle fatigue. If you work out too much, you can create temporary weakness. But if you don't work out at all, your muscles can atrophy (waste away)—which can also cause fatigue. This situation is called deconditioning.

Energy Conservation Strategies: Move—but pace it. Make sure you provide yourself with plenty of five-to-ten minute rest periods in between activities. Even if you feel pain when you walk, or you feel too weak to move, or your spasticity makes movement difficult, consult a therapist and keeping trying! Staying mobile, even for short bursts of time, is crucial. If walking is too difficult and you need to use a wheelchair, make sure that you do range-of-motion exercises with the help of your physical therapist to avoid atrophy.

Be "activity tolerant": Break down a specific activity into small steps that you can perform easily and make time for rest. For example, if you wanted to clean your house:

- Choose only one job per day and alternate, say, vacuuming the bedroom carpet with dusting off your night table.
- Keep a basket or pail full of cleaning supplies that you can carry with you from room to room—instead of having to walk up and down the stairs to get a can or bottle or rag.
- Use adaptive equipment specifically designed to make life easier: long extended handles on dusters, brushes, and mops; lightweight Dustbusters® and vacuums; kneeler/seat combinations; stools; and easy-to-maneuver scooters with baskets. These will help you avoid any unnecessary movement that can cause fatigue.

Tiring Trouble #3: "I Feel Sleepy" or Biochemical Lassitude

There are times when everybody wants to take a nap. But for people with MS, the sudden, overwhelming sleepiness that comes over them can be a dangerous handicap. This lassitude, as it is called, may occur abruptly and severely, any time of day or night.

Lassitude is also frustrating because a person can look so good, so healthy, that no one would ever think there was a problem. It's an "invisible" symptom—until it strikes. This can cause trouble for both the person with MS and those around her. Rather than go through detailed explanations and face the possible "pity" or confusion in the eyes of others, a person with MS might hide the fact that she has this disease. The people around her might get angry: Why can't she go to the movies? She looks fine! What's her problem? It must be in her head. . . ." Or worse, they might smother her with love and devotion, treating her like an invalid who needs to stay in bed.

Energy Conservation Strategies: Because lassitude is most likely a biochemical reaction to a brain lesion, medications that affect the chemistry of the brain can help. These include:

- *Amantadine hydrocholoride:* An antiviral medication that is also used for Parkinson's disease. Four clinical studies have found that 100 mgs taken twice a day can help reduce general fatigue.
- *SSRI antidepressants (Prozac®, Zoloft®):* These antidepressants not only help balance the chemical serotonin in your brain and help lift your depression, they also give you energy. (Some people experience flu-like symptoms with SSRIs, but the energizing effect far outweighs any side effects.)
- *Modafinil (Provigil®):* This is a fairly new medicine, one that has been used successfully in people with narcolepsy (excessive daytime sleepiness), brain injury, and stroke. An Ohio State University study found that 200 mgs every day significantly decreased fatigue.
- *Methylphenidate (Ritalin®):* This drug, now synonymous with ADD (Attention Deficit Disorder), is safe and well tolerated by people of all ages. Studies show that it helps people "wake up" during the day; it also has the added plus of improving attention span and concentration.
- *Pemoline (Cylert®):* Although a central nervous system stimulant, this medication is not an amphetamine. Its

properties are similar to Ritalin® and it has been used successfully in people who have ADD.

In addition to medicine, lassitude can be controlled with a few life strategies: frequent rest periods, planned naps, and proper pacing throughout the day.

Tiring Trouble #4: "Stressed Out, Anxious, and Depressed" or The Psychological Link

Depression can be an insidious condition. In addition to being a terrible disease in its own right, depression can also be a symptom of many other diseases, including MS. *(See Chapter 12 for in-depth information on depression.)* And one of its most characteristic factors is fatigue. Think about it: hopeless and helpless feelings can make anyone tired—especially someone who is predisposed to have fatigue.

Further, the stress of coping with multiple sclerosis and the anxiety it brings to the party can also create fatigue. Worrying can be an aerobic exercise for the mind. All the fussing and fuming, all that free-floating fear, all the very real things that are happening to you and your body—these thoughts can make you very tired.

And, to add insult to injury, the depression and anxiety might interrupt your sleep. You'll go around exhausted all day long—fueling the fatigue that's already there. *(Sleep patterns can also be altered by bladder problems, specifically a need to urinate during the night. We'll be going over this particular symptom in Chapter 13.)*

Energy Conservation Strategies: The best defense is an offensive—in this case, the same SSRI antidepressants that are used for lassitude. Not only will you treat your fatigue, but your underlying depression as well. And, because studies have shown that depression is best treated by a combination of medicine and counseling, we advise you to seek out a therapist in your MS center or ask your doctor or nurse for a referral.

Stress-reducing activities can help as well: Yoga, meditation, and deep breathing can all go far in reducing your stress levels. *(Read about more stress-reducing strategies in Chapter 12.)*

PILL TALK

Another source of fatigue that is often discounted is the side effects of the medication you are taking. Some of the medications used in the treatment of MS can cause fatigue in some people. Some antidepressants can make you sleepy. Talk to your doctor. Make sure she is aware of all the pills you take every day.

Tiring Trouble #5: "I Think, Therefore I am" or Cognitive Problems

If your thoughts are cloudy, it seemingly takes a long time to think or make a decision, you can't remember things, you find yourself reading the same words over and over, you have trouble paying attention—these are all problems with your cognitive ability. They occur when myelin and axonal deterioration occurs in your brain. And not only are they problems in their own right, they can be exhausting! In other words, cognitive problems can leave you fatigued.

Memory loss is the most common cognitive problem seen in people who have MS. Very simply, memory is defined as the function in the brain that registers, consolidates, and, later, retrieves information. That information is selective and unique to each person. It is based on what he sees, what he reads, what he thinks. If the memory process is interrupted by myelin damage anywhere along this register-retrieve continuum, there may be some temporary or permanent loss.

Short-term and long-term memory depend on different circuits in the brain—and short-term memory difficulty is the one experienced by people with MS. Some can remember the past quite clearly, but cannot remember the name of someone they've known only a few months.

It is the terrible poignancy of this problem, the frustrating and hurtful forgetfulness that, more than anything else, can make MS so difficult on family members and friends. Along with memory loss, a person with MS can also suffer from an inability to focus on the task at hand; he can have problems with attention and information processing; she can become depressed, anxious, and very, very tired.

The worst problem? Even subtle memory loss can affect a person's ability to work. If she cannot remember how to access a file in her computer, she will make mistakes in her reports. If he cannot remember how to appraise a used car, his boss may worry about his ability to sell it later on.

Although approximately 40–60% of all people who have MS will suffer some cognitive difficulties, only 10% have severe problems. For the majority of people, cognitive problems are annoying, frustrating, and fatiguing. They may have some problems with memory and information processing, but they are also capable of brilliant thoughts and action.

Energy Conservation Strategies: Memory training concentrates on practical solutions rather than on memory improvement alone. As in all aspects of rehabilitation, there is great overlap, and speech and language pathologists will work in concert with occupational therapists on memory impairment. With this in mind, after careful testing and evaluation, a rehabilitation team will use a variety of techniques to retrain a brain. They include:

- *Memory notebooks.* These notebooks are individual "appointment books" that help organize your life. They show you what to do and when to do it. Here are the names, descriptions, and places that are important to you. Here, too, are your daily schedules, your rehabilitation activities, your lunch dates, your shopping lists, your important birthdays and holidays—even your rehabilitation progress reports. Whenever your memory fails, you simply turn to your notebook to get the answers you need. In today's high-tech world the memory notebook has been replaced by the Palm Pilot® or similar devices. If you have trouble writing, some of these even have voice-recognition features.

- *Mnemonics.* Although they sound serious, these are actually a series of games. They trigger memories by associating visuals, puns, or silly slang to a word, a phrase, or a proper name. "Nana Anna ate a banana" is a mnemonic; it would trigger a relative's name in your mind. Picturing Hungary on a map of the world would help you think of the word hungry when you wanted dinner. It could also stimulate an appetite that's been waylaid by a lesion.

CHAIN OF COMMAND

Think about the 13 steps it takes to make a peanut butter and jelly sandwich to have with a glass of milk and some chips. You:

1. *Must find peanut butter and jelly on shelf of refrigerator and move them to the counter.*
2. *Must get a knife out.*
3. *Must get a loaf of bread out of the pantry.*
4. *Must get a plate and glass out of the cupboard.*
5. *Must get milk out of the refrigerator.*
6. *Must get chips out of the pantry.*
7. *Must get a napkin out.*
8. *Must put peanut butter on bread.*
9. *Must put jelly on bread.*
10. *Must put two pieces of bread together.*
11. *Must put milk in the glass.*
12. *Must put peanut butter and jelly and milk back into refrigerator.*
13. *Must put dishes in the sink when finished eating.*

Written out like this, making a sandwich becomes a big production! But for someone with memory loss, this "chain of commands" can be a lifesaver: It can make the difference between being dependent on others or living an independent life. Worked out and "rehearsed" with your occupational therapist, the steps in this activity will be easy for you to follow—especially if drawers and cabinets are labeled and your kitchen is clean and quiet. Eventually, your memory might be stoked back to life—and you'll remember how to make your sandwich without referring to the list.

- *Consistent Environment.* There's nothing like a calm, clean, quiet environment to help reduce *anyone's* stress levels. But if you have memory problems, this consistent, structured, and safe environment does even more: It can help give you the focus and calmness to help you retrieve that word, that name, that holiday, that you'd forgotten.
- *Organized Items.* If you have memory problems, it helps to always keep things in the same place: keys on the hook by the front door, glasses in the cabinet over the sink, tee-shirts and underwear in the top drawer of your bureau. Labeling each drawer and cabinet can also help trigger your memory.
- *Lists and More Lists.* Although you might keep daily logs in your memory notebook, it helps to keep a pad and pencil handy, ready for you to jot down any thoughts as they occur to you—from the supplies you need at the drugstore to the phone calls you need to return. And always keep your pad and pencil in the same place!
- *Mind Games.* Keep your brain stimulated and your mind active with puzzles, computer games, surfing the web, or board games. Think of them as "brain aerobics." You're exercising your body, why not your mind? But again, don't push past the point of fatigue. As soon as you find your fun factor dissipating and your mind a' wandering, stop.

Tiring Trouble #6: "Ouch! That hurts!" or Pain

Pain is so general a symptom of multiple sclerosis that it is often overlooked. Many times, physicians will connect pain to a different disease—or they will consider it "all in your head." But the fact is that 80% of people who have MS, both relapsing-remitting and progressive, suffer from some form of pain; 15% of them suffer from chronic pain that doesn't go away—and 20% suffer so much that it interferes with their activities of daily life. Although we are not sure of the reason, more women than men experience pain.

Why pain? Because MS creates a malfunction in the central nervous system's ability to "close the door" on painful sensations. The result is a surge of literally sensational information which cannot be controlled. Some of the problems that are created include:

- **Paresthesias,** or numbness and a tingling sensation. It is the same feeling you get when your arm "falls asleep" at night and needs a few quick shakes to be revived.
- The same malfunction is at the root of **dysesthesias,** a strange hot, burning, or even electric-shock like sensation that is basically a more much painful paresthesias. It can be so bad that people cannot bear to wear clothes against their skin.
- **Neuralgia** is pain along a specific nerve passageway—especially the sharp, painful electrical shocks to the face caused by *trigeminal neuralgia* along the 5th cranial nerve.
- **L'hermitte's sign** is another sharp, sometimes painful electrical shock, this time felt down your back when you bend your neck forward. L'hermitte's sign is a result of myelin damage in the neck region of your spinal cord. *(See Chapter 4 for detailed information on these and other symptoms of MS.)*

Pain can also be the result of physical symptoms. The tight, clenched muscles in spasticity can cause a "Charley horse", a cramp-like type of pain. *(See chapter 10 for a full explanation of and treatment for spasticity.)* An improper gait or balance difficulties can create cramps, aches, and swollen knees or ankles; lower back pain, although not a direct symptom of MS, can become a chronic problem because of overcompensation. An MS-related walk or stance may put additional stress on the spine—aggravating any co-existing arthritis or disc degeneration. *(See Chapter 2 for information on the anatomy of the spine.)*

Pain can also be emotional. When you are depressed, you may feel aches, cramps, and constant pain in your joints, muscles, and tendons. Further, your emotional torment can make you less tolerant of any pain you experience.

Energy Conservation Strategies: There is hope for pain—and its name is medicine. But not your usual aspirin or acetaminophen or prescription painkillers. *Your pain is*

PAIN BY ANY OTHER NAME

When you are feeling pain, it may seem like nothing else matters. But scientists, researchers, and physicians have taken "pains" to learn more about it. Pain has been studied and analyzed; it can be categorized into two types. Paroxysmal pain starts suddenly and randomly; it is intermittent. It is a sharp, jolting pain that tends to come and go; it can last anywhere from only a few seconds to a few hours. Chronic pain is any pain that lasts longer than six months despite multiple attempts at treatment.

not the result of injury or surgery—and traditional pain medication will be less effective at best, and addictive at worst.

Some of the drugs that have been successful in treating nerve pain include:

- *Carbamazepine (Tegretol®)* calms down short-circuited, "jumpy" sensory nerves—although doctors and researchers aren't sure why or how it works. Initially given in small doses, this medication eventually builds up in your system to the point where it controls your pain. An extended release form similar to carbamazepine called oxycarbamazepine (Carbatrol® and Trileptal®) is also available; it doesn't have to be taken as frequently—only twice a day.

- *Phenytoin (Dilantin®)* also calms down nerves along your sensory passageways, but it tends to work for only a small number of people.

- *Gabapentin (Neurontin®)*, an antiepileptic drug, is one of the most effective drugs in helping the burning pain of dysesthesias. It has also been found to ease the pain of migraine headaches in some patients. The dose can vary greatly; some patients receive high dosages (90 mgs—3,600 mgs).

- *Amitriptyline (Elavil®)* is an antidepressant, but it has also been found to be effective in altering the "pain" message that goes to the brain. It is best taken at bedtime since it makes many people drowsy.

- *Diazepam (Valium®)* is a muscle relaxer and can be used for spasticity, spasms, and back pain. However, it should be used sparingly because it can affect cognition and become habit-forming.

- *Capsaicin cream (Axsain®, Zostrix®)* may help with dysesthesias pain. It can be bought over the counter in a .075% concentration.
- *Ibuprofen (Motrin®, Advil®)* and naproxen (*Naprosyn®, Aleve®*) are non-steroidal anti-inflammatory drugs (NSAIDs) that can be purchased over the counter. They can help with chronic back pain, headaches, and joint pains.

And don't underestimate the power of exercise. Performing range-of-motion stretches to a point *before* fatigue can help ease back and muscle pain. (Remember: strength-training exercises don't work for some people with MS. It just makes them weaker and causes them to tire that much sooner. Check with your doctor and therapist to see what exercises are right for you.) Speak to your physical therapist about adaptive equipment that can make walking less painful. Massage and the application of heat can also help back pain.

This ends our "sleepover" portion of our journey. But there are still two more common symptoms that must be explored. . . .

CHAPTER TWELVE

FIGHTING DEPRESSION: MS AND YOUR EMOTIONAL HEALTH

"But you look so good!" That's what people say to me
all the time. If they only knew how bad I feel inside.
If they only knew I was really depressed.
If they only knew how tough it is sometimes
to put on a happy face.

—A 36-year-old news reporter with MS
who has just started treatment for depression

No one could say that Marlene was lazy. As a single mom with a three-year-old toddler, an aging mother, and a "deadbeat" dad who paid child support only sporadically, she had her hands full. She had no time to sleep, let alone meet another man. And when you add the fact that she lived up to every penny she got from her job as a seamstress for a famous designer—a job she loathed—you can practically see the stress steaming out from her head.

Marlene's life situation alone would be reason enough for her to be depressed. But there was also a history of depression in her family—which made Marlene more vulnerable to the ups and downs of life.

One night, after a full day of pinning and sewing for the designer's upcoming fall fashion show, Marlene came home with one of her horrible migraines. She had felt it coming on all day. It was so intense she needed to lie down; she called her neighbor and asked her to watch her daughter; she didn't check the answering machine to see if her mother had called. She closed her eyes. . . .

But Marlene couldn't sleep. In addition to the splitting migraine headache, she started feeling numb on one side of her face. She was nervous, scared. What if she was having a stroke? It wasn't impossible in 36-year-old women.

The next day Marlene's headache was gone—but the numbness remained. She called in sick at work and went to see her doctor. He examined her and couldn't find anything physically wrong, but there was no mistaking her depression: Her stance, her sloppy clothes, her lack of focus and energy—all were signs of depression. The doctor prescribed an antidepressant for her depression.

Marlene went back to work and her routine went back to normal. She was so busy that she didn't realize it at first, but—yes—the numbness was gone! It had been about three days since she'd gone to the doctor and started taking the antidepressant so it had to be "all in her head."

But three months later, the numbness came back—along with a slight blurring of her vision. This time, her doctor referred her to a neurologist. Maybe her symptoms were not psychological.

The neurologist gave Marlene a thorough examination; she asked Marlene all sorts of questions about her background and family history. She had Marlene undergo an MRI—which came back normal. The neurologist shook her head: Marlene seemed perfectly fine. The numbness and tingling sensations must be side effects of her migraine headaches. She told Marlene to continue taking her antidepressant and recommended that she go into therapy.

Marlene was relieved—but still concerned. She didn't have the time or money to see a therapist. She was fine; she just needed some time off. The antidepressants were expensive to boot. She finished them and then threw the bottle away. It was time for a clean slate. Marlene was strong and capable— the neurologist even said she was healthy. She didn't need medication!

A year went by. Marlene's daughter had left the "terrible twos" behind and she'd found an affordable assisted-living home for her mother. Even her job was going smoothly. For the first time in years, Marlene had time to take a breath.

But not for long. Suddenly, while Marlene was working, her hands started to shake. Not a lot, but enough for her to notice that her usually perfect hems were coming out a bit crooked. Marlene also found herself squinting at her stitches.

Marlene found herself back in her neurologist's office; the doctor repeated the MRI which came out normal. Once again, Marlene admitted to being under too much stress. How can she work if she couldn't sew a straight seam! The neurologist told Marlene to start taking her antidepressants again; she stressed the importance of seeing a therapist.

Unfortunately, Marlene was stubborn—and so depressed that she didn't think anything would help, let alone a therapist and a couple of pills! She went back to work and, during the next six months, she tried to ignore her symptoms— which now included a lack of coordination in her hands when she sewed. But when Marlene started seeing double— two needles, two threads—she knew it couldn't be in her head. Something had to be wrong.

Depressed and scared, Marlene went back to her neurologist. This time the MRI did not come back normal. The neurologist told Marlene that she had multiple sclerosis. Multiple sclerosis?! How could that be! Marlene was furious. Why didn't her doctor tell her that two and a half years ago?

Marlene was so angry that she went to another neurologist—who told her the same thing: she had MS. It could not have been diagnosed until now, until her MRI came back abnormal. There was no way her doctor could have discovered the truth; there was no one to blame. In fact, five percent of people who have MS start out with normal MRIs.

Although Marlene realized that she couldn't point fingers, that there was nothing anyone could have done until now, she became more and more depressed. It wasn't fair. She had too much going on her life, too much to handle. How could she raise her daughter? How could she do her job? How could she ever have an intimate relationship?

Marlene's depression spiraled down until she couldn't even get out of bed. She was in trouble—and she knew that, in addition to her new disease-modifying medication, she had to take her antidepressants. She had to start seeing a therapist.

Perhaps Marlene had depression in her genes. Perhaps her stressful life triggered it. Perhaps it would have gone away on its own. Or perhaps it was an actual MS symptom. None of that mattered. Marlene had the disease and she had to learn how to deal with it. She had to learn that depression was a normal symptom of MS—as was the confusion and conflicting emotions that come into play. Which came first, the chicken or the egg? It didn't matter. Marlene was depressed, and she needed help.

Marlene got the help she sorely needed—but not everyone is as fortunate. When an episode of MS strikes, it leaves a myriad of symptoms in its wake. And many of them are emotional. . . .

LIFE SIGNS: THE SIX STAGES THAT LEAD TO ACCEPTANCE

A person's emotional life is complicated enough without a disease or condition. The rites of passage, the stages we all go through, birth, death, marriage, divorce, the good times along with the sad, make for quite a ride. Add a disabling disease, however, and the equation immediately gets more complicated.

By its very definition, multiple sclerosis is not "happy." Let's face it: you don't order MS on the Internet. You don't want it, you don't want to go near it, you want it to go away— but you're stuck with it. Perhaps you'll lash out at your neurologist, like Marlene did, unable to accept the fact that your MS was not diagnosed sooner. Perhaps you'll be filled with despair, falling into a deep depression because of your disease. Or perhaps you'll deny there's anything wrong.

All these different responses are perfectly normal. In fact, in order to be mentally more healthy, many people go through six different stages when they hear they have MS. You too have to go through a grieving process before you can accept the fact that you have MS. However, it's important to keep in mind that the erratic nature of MS means that these stages may stop and start, some might be skipped, or some or all of them might be experienced in different ways.

Psychologist Elisabeth Kübler Ross first delineated her landmark six stages of grief in a discussion of terminal illness. But she could very well have applied them to any terrible shock—from the tragedy of 9/11 to a diagnosis of MS. The six stages of emotions that both you—and your loved ones— will experience at diagnosis and throughout the disease's course are:

Emotional Stage #1: "There's absolutely nothing wrong with me" or Denial

The shock at finding you have MS has a purpose: It hides the personal losses and the changes that may or may not come. When you first hear the news, you can often feel a sense of unreality, a sense that this could not be happening to you. Your brain simply cannot accept the fact that things have changed, that your life has changed—and that your disease may get worse over time.

Emotional Stage #2: "You're crazy, doctor! This just isn't fair!" or Anger

As the shock of the MS diagnosis wears off, anger sets in. "This is ridiculous," you might be thinking. "What did I do to deserve this!" You might kick something or lash out at someone you love. This stage can have a mixture of denial as well, a feeling that, "Hey, this is nothing. By next Spring, my symptoms will have disappeared and I will be as good as new!" Your loved ones, too, will feel anger as their relationships with you change, as they are forced to learn to accept the fact that your symptoms may get worse over time. They may be overwhelmed, afraid of the responsibility that has fallen on them; they, too, may lash out in anger.

Emotional Stage #3: "Listen, God, take away the MS and I will never, ever complain about anything again" or Bargaining

The shock is wearing off. Injecting one of the ABC + R drugs is becoming second nature. Your rehabilitation process has begun. You may find yourself praying, hoping, doing a lot of wishful thinking. Your loved ones, too, may find themselves bargaining with God, hoping against unrealistic hope that things will go back to the way they were.

Emotional Stage #4: "I will never be the same. I might as well give up" or Depression

Reality sets in. You may never be the same. Your life certainly will never be the same. The fact that you have MS will always be there; you will always wonder when—and if—the next episode will show up. Your relationships may be irrevocably changed; you may be treated differently. The old self, your old, healthier self, must be mourned. Some people, especially those whose symptoms continue to get worse, think about suicide. They want to give up—which makes them not only depressed, but overwhelmed with feelings of guilt as well. And their loved ones, tired of their caregiving role and just as guilty about their own ambivalent feelings, may also go through a depression. *(In fact, depression is so important an issue in MS that this chapter is specifically focused on it.)*

Emotional Stage #5: "Okay. It's real. I know it's real. I can't change it" or Acceptance

It is only when these feelings of depression, of guilt and anger, are dealt with that acceptance and healing can begin. Acceptance lies in the rational realm; it is knowing that things will be different, but that they still can work. Your medicine regimen and your rehabilitation are in full swing and your motivation is improving.

***Emotional Stage #6: "My God, I just laughed. I had
a good time. Maybe I can have a full life after all!"
or Hope***

From the depths of despair comes hope. Not the unrealistic
hope that you will never have an episode of MS again, but a
real hope, a valid hope that states, "There is value in who I am.
I am alive. Maybe I do have to alter my routine, but so what?
There is still a chance to live a full, happy, and satisfying life."

Not everyone goes through these six stages of emotions,
and not everyone goes through them in the same order. And,
unfortunately, these six stages are especially insidious if you
have MS because things can seem better after a flare-up. You
can have new symptoms for a few days or a few months—
and then nothing for a long time. It's easy to deny your disease—or believe that your "bargaining with God" has paid
off. Worse, when you do have another episode, it can throw
you for a loop—triggering feelings of hopelessness that were
already there, waiting in the wings; it can cause you to blame
yourself for not fighting hard enough.

You will experience these stages throughout the disease's
course, as your condition stabilizes, as symptoms flares up
again. Good, solid, supportive rehabilitation can go far in
helping you not only to move through these six stages, but
also to reach your goals—whatever they may be.

THE PSYCHOLOGICAL ASPECTS OF MS

It's easy to define a tremor or a problem with your gait or balance; these physical symptoms are visible. Even symptoms
such as optic neuritis, numbness, memory loss, and fatigue
can be easily described to your doctor or therapist. But there

are some symptoms that are not as noticeable; they can even be invisible—to both you and the outside world.

These are the psychological problems that a person with MS may face. They are not unique to MS; they are problems that many people with disabilities face. Let's go over some of these "psychological realms" now:

Psychological Realm #1: "Home Alone" or Social Isolation

Some people get anxious when they have to leave their house; some people are very shy and still others are more reclusive by nature.

This social isolation is a big problem for people with MS. They might be depressed because they've just been diagnosed. Their spasticity or weakness may make them too embarrassed to go out into the world, especially in their brand-new scooters. Their fatigue might motivate them to stay under the covers rather than going out and having to explain why they have to leave early. Whatever the reason, the more a person with MS isolates herself the more likely she will become depressed.

And that depression feeds on itself: You don't want to go anywhere. You don't want to see anyone and you don't want the phone to ring. You don't want to have fun, in fact, you can't.

Without help, your world will begin to shrink; your sense of community won't go any further than your TV. The "stay-at-home syndrome" can be potent indeed.

Solutions—Not Delusions: Get dressed every day. Shave or put on your makeup. Force yourself to go out at least once a day. If you can't seem to find the motivation, ask a friend, family member, or community aide to literally move you through the front door. (Perhaps you can even do some of your stretches and range-of-motion exercises in the Great Outdoors!) Medications for anxiety and depression can also help. *(We'll be discussing these in more depth later in the chapter.)*

Psychological Realm #2: "Money Talks" or Economic Strain

MS can be an expensive disease. Not only are the diagnostic tools and treatments costly, but you might also have to quit your job and do something else—which can translate into a reduction in salary.

Money problems are very stressful for even the healthiest person. Add MS and the problems can seem monumental. When you are fatigued, weak, or have difficulty in walking, you might not be able to handle a part-time job to help with the bills; you might not have the stamina.

Solutions—Not Delusions: The good news is that most health insurance providers will pick up the cost of at least a portion of your medicines, your MRIs, and rehabilitation therapy. To avoid unnecessary economic strain, speak to your case manager, your doctor, or the National Multiple Sclerosis Society. (1-800-FIGHT MS)

Psychological Realm #3: "Family Crisis" or Disruption of the Family Circle

The family is the most basic, life-sustaining structure in society. The bond within a family is strong, and as anyone who has family problems knows, its ties are felt even if that bond is weakened. Because of this primal, almost instinctual, bond, there is an unconscious striving to maintain order, or balance, within the family. This "law and order" is maintained via an unspoken hierarchy, or pecking order, in which everyone has his role, everyone has his place. There might be one or two breadwinners, a nurturing caregiver, a teased younger sibling, even a scapegoat. As long as everybody knows her role (usually on an unconscious level), peace is maintained and life in the family remains on an even keel.

But when the structure is disrupted, balance is lost. Tension and discord reign. Change, after all, threatens the continuation of the primal group, and it will be fought on both conscious and unconscious levels.

As you well know, MS brings change. Its consequences can be highly disruptive and fraught with tension—especially if the MS symptoms are severe and if they occur in the "leader of the pack", the one who rules the roost.

The result? Stress and its accompanying emotions come right in through the front door. Until a new hierarchy shifts into place, until new balance is attained, the family players may feel a "double dose" of anger, confusion, depression, and anxiety: one dose for the person they love who now has MS—and another one for themselves.

Solutions—Not Delusions: In a phrase: Families need therapy and guidance, too. Although the focus remains on the person who has MS, the family is a vital element, both for his recovery and for a return to a happy home. Families, too, need counseling to understand and cope with their own feelings of grief, fear, and anxiety. They need to understand their anger and their subsequent guilt. They need to restructure family balance and identity. They need to deal with the changes MS has brought to *everyone*. A good MS rehabilitation center always has a counselor and case manager to work with the family. And the National MS Society has information and programs to facilitate coping.

Psychological Realm #4: "Subtle Signs" or the Ambiguity of MS

One of the main frustrations of MS is its unpredictability. Even when you have been diagnosed with the disease, your uncertainty remains. You are always aware of your symptoms, monitoring them, and waiting for the "other shoe to drop." Your MS may improve to the point where it feels like a distant memory—or it may suddenly get worse when you least expect it. You'll never know.

MS can also take years to diagnose. Like Marlene in our scenario at the beginning of this chapter, you might find yourself overwhelmed and angry when you finally learn you have MS. For others, getting the diagnosis is a relief; the mystery of their fatigue, weakness, and double vision has been solved.

Solutions—Not Delusions: The best way to handle the ambiguity of MS is with the Scouts' motto: Be prepared. Your doctor and your therapist should be there to educate you up front and early on in your disease. They should tell you about symptoms you may not yet (or never!) experience, as well as offer strategies to cope with them. Finding out as much information about MS as you can will help you in the future. It's like a savings account: You may never need to use it, but it's there.

Being prepared can also help you in making life decisions. Perhaps you'll buy a ranch-style house instead of a split-level. Maybe you'll delegate some of your work on the job. And maybe you will find that joining a gym or going to a nutritionist is much less a luxury than a real necessity for your health.

Psychological Realm #5: "The Primal Scream" or Stress, Stress, and More Stress

We all experience stress in our lives. It's the nature of living in this hectic information age. Not only do we learn about catastrophes within minutes, but our own lives move much faster than they did in generations past. We can't get rid of stress; we just need to know how to handle it.

This is especially true with MS. Some people think there is a definite link between stress and the worsening of their MS symptoms. Others believe that learning how to cope with stress can reduce them.

However, science doesn't back this up. Although a few studies have shown a *possible* link between the growth of lesions in MS and stress, scientists are not yet convinced. Does a stressful event trigger MS? Can lesions influence the way we handle stress? Studies of this issue have been inconclusive. No one yet knows for sure and it is important we don't jump to unfounded conclusions

What we do know is that in times of stress many people with MS seem to have more symptoms—and they are reduced when the stressful situation goes away.

Most likely, this is the result of the nature of stress itself. When a person feels stressed and anxious, it takes much more energy to think, solve problems, or plan. On the other hand, take away the stressful situation—and the mind calms down. Cognitive abilities become clearer and take less energy. Life becomes easier again.

But how do you "take the stress away"? It might seem as if the stress itself influences your MS symptoms, but in reality, it is *the way you cope* with that stress that makes all the difference. You can't always change a stressful situation. But you can change the way you deal with it.

Solutions—Not Delusions: The first thing you must do is recognize stress—which can be easier said than done if you have MS. The same symptoms of stress—fatigue, tight muscles, weakness, numbness, tremors—are similar to the ones for MS. If you have been under a lot of pressure lately, if you've been anxious or depressed, chances are your symptoms are, at least in part, the result of stress. (The stress can also make them appear exaggerated.)

Once you've realized that you are stressed out, you have to identify the cause: is it work-related? Personal? Who is involved? Only then can you do something about it. Our body tells us to relocate, leave, or flee the stressful environment. But that is not usually an option. Most of the time, we have to learn how to cope with it. Some suggestions:

- *Deep breathing exercises or meditation.* Even five minutes of calm can reduce your stress levels. Studies have found that meditation can lower high blood pressure.
- *Gentle yoga moves.* Like meditation, the stretches you do in yoga provide a calm haven. (Make sure to check with your doctor about doing yoga or any exercise.)
- *Journal writing.* There's nothing like a blank book to pour out your frustrations and anger. Keeping a diary not only helps you recognize stress, but allows you to unleash it through words.
- *Biofeedback.* This device helps you monitor your stress-induced emotions via your physiology: heart rate, respiratory changes, and body temperature.
- *Talk.* The ideal situation would be talking to the person who caused you the stress. If that's not possible, try a

good conversation with a sympathetic ear: a close friend, a family member, your therapist, or the members of your support group.

Psychological Realm #6: "Sing it High, Sing it Low, or Mood Swings

Mood swings. The elation of a high, the depths of despair in a low. People who have MS are vulnerable to abrupt changes in mood. You might cry at the drop of a hat. You might laugh in the middle of a concert. These swift changes in mood can be a result of your disease: MS lesions can create structural changes in your brain—which may affect your brain chemistry and your mood.

There is another reason: the powerful steroids you take when you have an acute attack. High-dose steroids have been found to produce anxiety, insomnia, and emotional lability in people.

It makes sense that these unpredictable mood swings can be stressful—to you and the people around you.

Solutions—Not Delusions: First things first: See your doctor. If the steroids are causing your mood swings, the dosage can possibly be changed. Further, he may prescribe additional medication to keep your moods in balance. Antidepressants, anti-seizure medicines, and anti-anxiety drugs have all been found to work successfully. Your therapist can also offer strategies to deal with your changeable moods. One note: Your needs may change as your disease progresses, so don't forget to check with your physician about possibly increasing or decreasing the dose—or whether you can actually taper off some of your medicines completely.

These psychological realms are all aspects of your emotions—whether or not you have MS. And each one of them can lead to depression—which, in people with MS, can become a serious threat.

ARE YOU DEPRESSED?

Most people who have MS will have episodes of depression—and then get over it. You don't have to be a rocket scientist to know that an attack is going to add stress and confusion to your life—at least when it is in full swing. You might feel weepy, sad, or irritable. You might have trouble sleeping. You might lose your desire or your ability to have sexual relations.

Usually, with time, the depression lifts on its own. Suddenly, without your doing a thing, you'll notice that, despite your MS, your mood is better, that you are beginning to smile again, that life has hope.

The trouble may start with subtle sadness—which isn't as easy to recognize. You might not even realize you are depressed—until it has taken hold. Its onset can have insidious results for people with MS. Maybe you'll stop using your particular ABC + R drug. Maybe you'll lose your motivation to do your exercises. Maybe you'll feel even more fatigued. Or maybe you'll just give up and stop your rehabilitation altogether.

This is when depression takes on a life of its own, sabotaging your good work, erasing your hope for the future, and zapping your energy. If you feel helpless and hopeless about your MS, unable to work or function on a day-to-day basis for more than two weeks, you might very well be depressed. The symptoms of depression include:

FOLLOW THE POSITIVE ROAD

It might sound like a cliché, a theory framed in smiley faces and white clouds, but if you think happy, you will be happy. It has been proven that positive thoughts beget more positive thoughts—and thinking positive thoughts is a skill you can acquire. This "learned optimism" is based on some very simple truths:

•Don't dwell on the things you cannot change. As difficult as it may seem, accept the fact that you have MS and go on. Ruminating about it will only cause more stress—and anxiety.

•Try to think of concrete solutions to problems you may have. If necessary, write down what's bothering you. Then step back for a moment and pretend you are only an observer. What would you do to change things? Maybe you need to add more adaptive equipment to your home environment. Maybe you need a new scooter. Or maybe you need some additional training in giving yourself an injection. Seeing your problems plainly, in black and white, will help you work out solutions.

- Excessive crying
- Extreme fatigue and lack of energy
- Excessive anxiety
- Inability to focus on the task at hand; unable to concentrate

- Social withdrawal from others
- Apathy toward people and activities
- Insomnia—or too much sleep
- Loss of appetite—or eating too much
- Extreme irritability; low boiling point
- Lack of joy in all things
- Loss of sexual feelings
- Rumination; obsessive thoughts
- Negative feelings, such as hopelessness and helplessness
- Irrational guilt
- Death thoughts including suicide
- Lack of self-esteem

If you exhibit at least five of these symptoms, you may not only have MS—but be clinically depressed. Seek help from your physician as soon as possible.

AND NOW THE GOOD NEWS

Despite the way it makes you feel, depression is not all gloom and doom. The fact is that there is help out there, solid, real help that can make you feel better quickly. These include:

- *Antidepressant Medication.* Depression may not just be a reaction to your MS. In fact, your MS may be the trigger for a depression that has been lying dormant all these years. Millions of people suffer from depression—and are genetically predisposed to succumb to it. Clinical depression has been linked to low levels of serotonin and norepinephrine, both neurotransmitters,

BEHIND CLOSED DOORS: SEXUAL FUNCTION, PART I THE THREE "R's"

*Sexual problems are common among people with chronic illness—but they are rarely talked about. Doctors shy away from the subject; patients are too embarrassed to talk. Even people without disease are affected by fatigue, stress, and work pressures. Why not you? Add the three "R"s—fear of **R**ejection, fear of **R**idicule, and the very powerful fear of a **R**elapse—and sexual feelings can disappear (along with your self-esteem and confidence!)*

If you are having difficulty with intimacy, talk to your partner. Share your feelings, learn to be flexible, and don't be afraid to discuss your problems with a therapist or family counselor. Some antidepressants cause sexual dysfunction; your doctor may be able to change your medicine or dosage.

Remember: Depression can be treated—and so can your sexual dysfunction.

in the brain; at these low levels, they are not properly metabolized, and messages at the brain's synapses become skewed. Depression is associated with abnormal brain chemistry. The depression is an expression of a chemical imbalance that should be addressed with medication. Antidepressants, particularly selective serotonin reuptake inhibitors (SSRI), have been found to alter the imbalance—not by increasing the level of serotonin in your brain, but by altering the way serotonin acts within the brain. When there is a change in the way serotonin works (or, in scientific terms, uptakes) at your synapses, your spirits are lifted and the symptoms of depression decrease. SSRIs are approximately 70% effective in clinically depressed people. Some brand names include Prozac®, Zoloft®, and Effexor®. Other antidepressants manipulate norepinephrine, another neurotransmitter that may be imbalanced when a person is depressed. Wellbutrin® is one of these more popular medications—with the added benefit of decreasing the craving for nicotine.

BEHIND CLOSED DOORS:
SEXUAL FUNCTION, PART II

Fear is only part of the sexual dysfunction story. In addition to psychological inhibitors, physical problems can also cause a dip in sexuality. MS symptoms, such as immobility, bladder dysfunction, and cognitive problems, as well as certain medications, can cause impotence in men and women. But there is help:

- *Studies have shown that Viagra® has helped 50% of men who have MS. Erections can also be enhanced with self-injections of Alprostadil.*
- *Vibrating cuffs can help men with sensory problems in the genital area.*

- *A vacuum tube and hand pump device, called vacuum tumescence constriction therapy (VTCT) can be used successfully by men who have MS. It actually "pumps" up the penis by providing pressure on the veins in the penis—which, in turn, fills the penis up with blood and creates an erection.*
- *Women who experience vaginal dryness can use lubrications such as KY Liquid® and Astroglide®.*
- *Medication can be helpful in treating some painful sensory disturbances in a woman's genital area.*
- *Spasticity problems can be eased with massage, cold packs, and medication.*
- *Fatigue can be alleviated with energy management programs and by having sexual activities when a person is most energetic. Some positions require less energy than others. Talk with your partner.*
- *Medications that cause sexual dysfunction can be changed—either in dosage, time when taken, or brand.*
- *Cognitive problems, such as forgetting when you last had sex or misinterpretation of your partner's actions, requires patience—and possible counseling*
- *Alternative sexual positioning, using pillows or a side position, can ensure less pain and discomfort, as well as more pleasure.*
- *Catheters can be secured so there are no embarrassing moments. Your doctor can show you how this is done.*

- *Talk Therapy.* Not only is one-on-one "talk" therapy crucial for antidepressants to be effective, it can also work well on its own. Psychiatrists, psychologists, and clinical social workers are all licensed to help you cope better with stress, grief, and life's daily ups and downs. Check with your family physician or the National Multiple Sclerosis Society *(see address in back of book)* for someone who specializes in the treatment of people with MS.

- *Family Therapy.* Remember: MS is a disease that affects everyone close to you. *(See the section on family dynamics earlier in this chapter.)* If your family members take care of themselves, they will be better able to help take care of you. Less stress for them means less stress for you. Family therapy counsels the whole family at one time and individually. A family therapist can help rid the anger, frustration, sadness, and guilt that fester inside each family member—including you. She can help restore equilibrium within the fold.

- *Antianxiety medication.* Sometimes depression comes with "excess baggage": worry, nervousness, obsessive thinking, compulsiveness, or, in a word: anxiety. If you find that your mind is going a mile a minute, that you are terrified of leaving the house, or that your accelerated thoughts are making you immobile, you might need more than an antidepressant to see you through. Antianxiety medication can help calm the fears, worries, and unpredictability of your MS that seem to haunt your days. Brand names include Valium®, Xanax®, Ativan®, and BuSpar®. *Caution: Antianxiety medications can make you drowsy. They can also be habit-forming and are best used for short periods of time. People with MS who require these medications for long periods should be closely monitored by their physicians.*

- *Cognitive therapy.* It might not sound exciting, but this short-term psychotherapy can work. Using logic, exercises, and "hands on" worksheets, this therapy helps decrease the irrational negative thinking that comes into play when you feel hopeless and helpless. Cognitive therapy techniques are often incorporated into other types of therapy.

- *Support groups.* Perhaps you're having trouble adjusting to your difficulties in walking. Perhaps you're embarrassed about your lack of bladder control. Or perhaps you hate the way people seem to pity you as soon as you tell them you have MS. Whatever the reason, you are not alone. The emotional upheaval you feel is shared by many other people who have multiple sclerosis—and there is a group of these people meeting in your neighborhood as you are reading this. Call 1-800-FIGHT MS, the National Multiple Sclerosis Society hotline, to find a support group that meets near you. *(See additional contact information in the back of this book.)* Support groups provide friendship, practical information, understanding and, yes, that much-needed support when you are diagnosed with MS.

- *Lifestyle changes.* It's not sexy. It's not glamorous. But it's true. A nutritious diet and a regular exercise program approved by your doctor can help keep your energy levels up and your spirits high. Studies show that:

√ **Exercise can work as an antidepressant**—and do a lot of other good things for your body, too. When you swim in a lukewarm pool or just stretch and walk for only ten minutes at a time, the chemical endorphin is released in the brain. This neurotransmitter is responsible for feeling good. The more endorphins released in your brain, the better you feel. They help stop pain and keep your mood up. Need another reason to exercise: It can help reduce your stress. Working your muscles will help stop you from worrying—and you'll also keep your weight on an even keel.

√ **Alcohol has a depressing** effect on your body. You might want that drink to keep your sadness at bay, but long term it will only make you feel worse. It can also interfere with your medication. Drink only in moderation.

√ **Caffeine and sugar can make your mood drop— fast.** That early morning coffee jolt might give you a "rush" initially, but by mid-afternoon the only "energy" you'll feel is a wallop of even more fatigue.

√ **Structuring your days is an asset.** Organizing your waking and sleeping patterns will help you stay focused; you'll be able to complete tasks in a timely fashion; your self-esteem will improve. It will also help if you have trouble sleeping or bladder and bowel concerns. How to get a routine that makes you happy? Pace yourself to avoid fatigue. Go to go to bed at the same hour every night and only use your bed as a place to sleep. And, as much as possible, keep your workload balanced. Strive for the middle ground: challenging, but not so much that it causes fatigue and stress-induced anxiety.

√ **Eating healthy foods has a healthy effect.** A low-fat, high-fiber diet will not only help you stay "regular", but it will help your heart stay strong and healthy. You will have much more energy than if you stuffed your face with high-fat desserts and fried foods. The fact that you have MS should not interfere with healthy eating habits. A poor diet will just add more problems. Although many special diets have been touted for MS patients, none are proven. Proceed with caution and consult your physician or dietitian.

√ **Optimism and positive thinking help heal.** This cannot be said often enough. You cannot underestimate how important a positive attitude is in avoiding depression. Try to always see the glass as half-full—not as half-empty.

THE MS PROFILE

You are not alone with your conflicting, confusing emotions. In fact, there is so much common ground that the National Multiple Sclerosis Society has put together an "MS profile" (adapted from the research of Dr. Nicholas LaRocca):

1. People with MS have the same psychological needs, reactions, and feelings as anyone else—and these needs are just as individual as each one of us.
2. This means that you will be distressed when you are first diagnosed—and you will feel extra stress and emotional upheaval with any exacerbations.
3. Your emotions, especially depression and anxiety, will fluctuate with the ups and downs of your MS.
4. You might experience a drop in self-esteem when you are first diagnosed—but studies show that most people

bounce back and maintain healthy self-esteem over the long haul, even when their symptoms get progressively worse.

5. If you have MS, you will probably be like the thousands of others who need and desire information about their disease. Most people with MS want to know as much as possible about it—especially any new research developments.

6. The physical symptoms of MS can bother you, but the psychological and cognitive symptoms, as well as coping with adaptations in daily living, play an equally important role.

You are not alone. You are not the only person out there with MS. You haven't been singled out. And, if you are depressed, welcome to the "club" that includes millions of others. There is help out there. You just need to ask for it.

Our journey through the symptoms of MS is almost at an end. But there is one more arena we must address, one that can create much embarrassment, low self-esteem, and, yes, depression. It's bladder and bowel problems and it's coming up next.

CHAPTER THIRTEEN

LIVING WITH BLADDER AND BOWEL DYSFUNCTION

*The most embarrassing moment I had was not falling
or being unable to hand a basket of rolls across the
table. It was not being able to control my bladder.
I'd feel a need to urinate, and before I could get to
the bathroom, out it came. I felt my cheeks getting
flushed; I knew my skirt would show a telltale
stain. More than anything, I wish my MS
hadn't left me with such a basic problem.
How can I feel like an adult?*

—A 58-year-old businesswoman
with secondary-progressive MS

Sam used to make fun of the laxative commercials on television. He laughed at the serious tone the actors took in the pharmacy aisles. He loved the ads that showed a couple (usually older) about to play golf, or go horseback riding, or play a round of tennis. Within seconds, the man or the woman would grimace; she couldn't go with him because of irregularity; he couldn't go because he was afraid he'd have to go out in the woods where toilets weren't available.

Sam laughed so hard he'd hit his knee; he'd talk back to the commercials, making fun of the actors' accents.

But that was when Sam was in his 30s—and before his multiple sclerosis had been diagnosed. Now, 20 years and several episodes later, Sam is no longer laughing. Regularity has become one of the major focuses of his life.

The problem sometimes was constipation. Not the kind that lasts a day or two, but constipation that didn't get better for weeks at a time. Sam once had to be hospitalized in order to remove impacted stool.

But as far as Sam was concerned, he had two problems: the constipation—and its accompanying bloat, gas, and cramps—and his terrible embarrassment.

Sam's self-esteem had already dropped when he first learned he had MS. And, with each relapse, it dropped a little more. Fortunately, he had the sense to go to a MS Rehabilitation Center. They knew how to help. And, unlike other clinics where the staff didn't want to discuss problems like constipation, the MS Center understood. The rehabilitation team understood that disruption in basic routines, such as bladder control and bowel movements, could hit people with MS harder than the fact that they couldn't walk. Without being able to control one's own bodily functions, independence is not possible. Add the feelings of embarrassment and very real discomfort, and people with MS—or any central nervous system disease—are hard pressed to find the motivation to get better.

Take Sam. Before he'd gone to the MS Center, he was sure he would never be independent. He was positive that he would have to live with his bloat and his gas. But the nurse at the Center not only talked to him about his constipation, she also provided strategies that would help him control his problem. A dietitian helped him get started on a fiber-rich diet. And the doctor-prescribed medicines that would ease his problem.

Sam was on his way: Thanks to his new regimen of disease-modifying drugs for his MS, antidepressants for his dropping self-esteem, and a complete program for his constipation, he felt in control, independent, and motivated.

And he never laughed at another irregularity commercial again. (But he still couldn't help himself when it came to frozen dinner ads.)

Irregularity. Constipation. Incontinence. Urinary tract infections. These words are all synonymous with embarrassment. A person who has problems with his bladder or his bowels has trouble being happy and completely independent. He has difficulty living a physically comfortable life.

MS Rehabilitation Centers know this—and that's why bladder and bowel functions (as well as swallowing—another basic function) are evaluated at the same time a person is learning to walk better.

This chapter will examine some of the successful strategies used for both bladder and bowel dysfunction—which occur in 50 to 90% of people with MS during the course of their disease.

But before you can determine the "cure", you need to know the why. . . .

THE LOW-DOWN ON ELIMINATION

Whether it's an apple or a pear, grilled salmon or soup, eventually all the food we eat is broken down into liquids. By the time food (now liquid) reaches our small intestines, it is further broken down into the most minute chemical components. Nutrients are absorbed by the body and utilized as cell food. Liquid waste is sent to the kidneys through the blood stream; solid waste travels through the large intestines for eventual elimination. *(We'll discuss solid waste and bowel problems later on in this chapter.)*

Basically, the kidneys act as filters, "cleaning" the blood and separating it even further—into life-sustaining fluids that are sent back through the bloodstream, as well as liquid waste that needs to be eliminated.

This liquid waste travels down thin tubes called ureters, one on either side of each kidney, to the bladder, where it is held until the urge to "go" passes it out through the urethra. (In men, the urethra is also the passageway for sperm.)

The pelvic muscles help keep waste where it belongs, in the bladder, until you're ready to relieve yourself. How do you know when to go? Enter the nervous system, which helps you determine when you can go—and when you need to hold it in. When the bladder gets full, a messenger is dispatched via the spinal cord to the brain, saying, "I'm uncomfortable!"

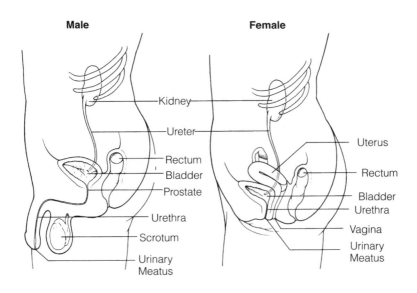

The Genitourinary System

The brain, in turn, tells your legs to get moving and find a bathroom fast. It also sends a message to the base of the spinal cord, where a group of nerves called the reflex arc initiate the actual voiding reflex "when the coast is clear." Bladder muscles then contract, pushing urine into the urethra and out of the body via the urethral sphincter. Aahh . . .

That's it. Different systems working together. Clear-cut, basic, and incredibly efficient—as long as the central nervous system is intact.

THE MS-URINARY TRACT CONNECTION

As you know now, MS lesions can appear anywhere in the central nervous system. When they affect the spinal cord pathways that connect the brain with the voiding reflex center, you may end up with some kind of urinary tract problem, or "bladder matter":

Bladder Matter #1: "Not Enough Space" or a Small Spastic Bladder

To help you understand this condition, let's go back to the urinary tract for a moment. The bladder muscles contract at a signal from the reflex arc at the base of your spine. As the bladder fills, the reflex action is to empty—regardless of where you are. Let's say you are driving in your car with a mugful of coffee inside you. Your bladder is definitely full. In people without MS (as well as in many people who do; it depends on the location of the lesions), the brain intervenes before you relieve yourself on the driver's seat. It would say, "Whoa. Hold it in. I see a rest stop up ahead . . ." Your brain would overrule the reflex arc and keep you full until you reached a bathroom. You might be uncomfortable, but you wouldn't be embarrassed.

When lesions affect the myelin in the spinal cord pathways between the reflex arc and the brain, there's no one in control. The reflex arc will automatically stimulate the full bladder to empty—no matter where you are. This is called a small spastic, or a failure to store, bladder.

Although not life-threatening, a small spastic bladder can make you feel like a toddler, unable to hold your urine. It is a difficult condition to accept because it involves your basic assumptions about being an adult.

Symptoms of a small spastic bladder may include:

- *Increased frequency of urination.* The times you urinate during the day can increase so much that you are voiding small amounts every 30 to 60 minutes.
- *Urgency.* You have the feeling, but not the control. Once you feel the urge to urinate, nothing can hold you back—literally. You may have trouble making it to the bathroom.
- *Dribbling.* This is exactly as it sounds: small amounts of urine are "leaked" from the bladder onto your underwear. Sometimes you may not even be aware of the leakage until you notice the dampness.
- *Incontinence.* This is one people with MS share with an aging population. Simply put, you cannot hold urine in your bladder; you don't reach the bathroom in time. Sometimes you may not even be aware of the need to urinate.

Bladder Matter #2: "Leftovers" or a Failure to Empty

When lesions appear in the base of the spinal cord, which directly affect the voiding reflex arc, your brain does not get appropriate messages. Nor does your bladder. The pathways to and from the brain and bladder are silent. Your bladder may fill to bursting, but you won't be aware of it. Nor can your bladder and sphincter get messages of control. They are just as out of touch as the brain. The result? An over-filled bladder that overfills again and again; you never completely void all of your urine. This is called failure to empty, or flaccid bladder.

Symptoms of this type of condition include the same frequency, urgency, incontinence, and dribbling that are found in a small spastic bladder. It also may include:

- *Hesitancy.* Often seen in people who have a urinary tract infection (UTI), hesitancy literally means a hesitant bladder. You have difficulty beginning to urinate, even though you have the urge. Hesitancy can be particularly uncomfortable because you can feel the urge to go—with no relief.

Bladder Matter #3: "Double Trouble" or Detrusor Sphincter Dysynergia

Think conflict and you'll understand this particular bladder problem. Your bladder's contractions cannot coordinate with your sphincter's reflex relaxing.

This is what happens if you have dysynergic or "conflicting" bladder:

1. Your bladder contracts, ready to release its urine . . .
2. . . . but the sphincter stays closed. This may result in both urgency and hesitancy.
3. A related problem: Your bladder relaxes, letting the urine fill it up . . .
4. . . . resulting in dribbling, or incontinence with retention of urine. This poses an increased risk of bladder infection and other urinary complications.

Because detrusor sphincter dysynergia can result in the backup of urine to the kidneys (particularly in men) and, ultimately, lead to kidney disease, it's important to talk to your doctor if you show any sign of a bladder problem.

OPEN BOOK TEST

A bladder program is essential to help avoid urinary tract infections, kidney failure or disease, and that quality of life-affecting embarrassment. In order to determine the extent of your bladder problems—as well as the progress you are making—your rehabilitation team, urologist (a specialist in the urinary tract) or neurologist will do one or more of these diagnostic "urination equation" tests:

Urination Equation Test #1: Urinalysis. This is the reason for the "little cup" when you go to the doctor's office. This test is the first step in determining preliminary conclusions about white blood cells in your urine (a sign of infection), possible diabetes, and more.

Urination Equation Test #2: Urine culture. This test may come from a "clean catch" specimen obtained while voiding or a non-contaminated specimen obtained by placing a catheter in your bladder. This specimen will be sent off to a laboratory where a culture will be "grown," determining if any bacteria are present. If your doctor suspects a urinary tract infection, she will also request a urine culture sensitivity; this will help determine which antibiotic will be the most effective to treat the infection.

Urination Equation Test #3: Intravenous Pyelogram (IVP). Don't worry: This is much less imposing than it sounds. In an IVP, your vein is injected with an iodine dye after a complete bowel elimination. An X-ray then traces a complete picture of the entire urinary system, including your kidneys, urethra, and bladder—to show your doctor if and where the problems lie.

Urination Equation Test #4: Cystometrogram. No, you won't be asked to pronounce it, but you should be aware of this test—it can be a crucial one for people with MS because it shows your doctor how your bladder reacts to filling up with urine. Saline, which mimics urine, is injected into your bladder. The result? Your doctor can determine if you have a spastic bladder (overactive) or a flaccid (under active) one. He can also see how much pressure builds up in your bladder before you need to void.

Urination Equation Test #5: Cystourethrogram. A cousin to the other unpronounceable test above, this one is an X-ray that utilizes dye (sent into the body via a catheter) to help your doctor see your bladder—its size, shape, and function.

Urination Equation Test # 6: Uroflowmeter. In this test you must drink fluids and fill up your bladder. You'll then urinate into a machine which determines the amount, intensity, and speed at which your urine flows.

Urination Equation Test #7: Cystoscopy. In some cases, a urologist might insert thin, snake-like tubes (smaller but still similar to those used in a colonoscopy to check your lower intestinal tract) into your bladder to look for narrowing of the urethra or thickening of the bladder wall.

Urination Equation Test #8: Post-Void Residual (PVR) Ultrasound. Like the sonar on submarines that detected enemy ships, this device, placed on the skin after voiding, actually uses sound waves to create a picture. As sound bounces back and forth on the tissue walls, an organ in the body is depicted on a monitor very similar to a TV screen. Although no Kodak moment, these pictures will help your doctor pinpoint any residual urine you might have in your bladder. Anything more than 100-150 ml. post-void residual (PVR) and you are at risk of getting a UTI.

Once your doctor knows the type of bladder problem you have—either flaccid, spastic, or dysynergic—a proper plan of action can be set. The main goals? Relieving symptoms, preventing accidents, and avoiding complications—such as repeating bladder infections—which risk your overall health.

Bladder problems may also fluctuate with the course of your disease. The good news is that there are very successful medicines and therapies that work. Let's go over them now:

CROSSING THE GREAT VOID: THE CATHETER

Catheterization is usually the treatment of choice if your bladder is not emptying all its urine when you try to urinate. It is a remarkable piece of simple engineering. The thin plastic tube is inserted into the bladder to drain urine. Period.

Although the device itself is simple, there are various types of catheterization. You might find one more convenient than another. Your urologist may feel one is more efficient than another. Whichever one is picked, it's not irrevocable. Your doctor can change the method if necessary.

ISC, or Intermittent Self-Cathertization, may be the first step in retraining your bladder. It is the program of choice if you have urinary retention and difficulty voiding. A catheter is placed in the bladder several times a day. There is a small opening at the end of the catheter tip; the other end of the tube has a larger opening. In most cares, urine will then flow out into the toilet. ISC can be done in any private place; your rehabilitation team will help you learn how to do it yourself. The same catheter can be reused after cleaning with soap and water. You'll be surprised how easy and comfortable this can be.

A Foley, or indwelling catheter, may be the best choice if you have no control at all. It remains in the bladder at all times, and it is changed every month to help keep infections at bay. Remember that when a catheter is left inside, there is a greater chance for infection. Cleanliness is crucial. In Foleys and other indwelling catheters, the end of the tube that is inserted holds a small balloon. This is filled with water or saline solution to keep the catheter in place inside of the bladder. The other end is connected to an external collection bag.

A suprapubic catheter is also left in the bladder and is used for the small group of people with MS whose bladder problems are not controlled by usual therapies. This device is placed directly into the bladder above the pubic bone via a small surgical incision in the abdomen. It is a good choice for people who get frequent infections.

External catheters are condoms that fit over a man's penis and are attached to a leg bag.

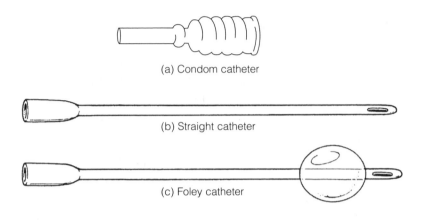

(a) Condom catheter

(b) Straight catheter

(c) Foley catheter

Catheters: (a) condom catheter which goes over the penis; (b) A straight rubber catheter for intermittent catheterization; (c) Foley catheterization with balloon

NO-NONSENSE RETRAINING: A VOIDING SCHEDULE AND JOURNAL

We might remember the slight embarrassment when we wet our pants as children. We might also remember that feeling of dread when we wet the bed. But remembering exactly when we were "potty trained" is not something we can easily bring to mind—even when we are training our own children.

That's why having to relearn bladder management can be emotionally difficult. But once you look at it rationally (with the help of a supportive rehabilitation team), you'll realize that urination is just another physical function. It just so happens that its automatic "on/off switch" has been disconnected or damaged. In most cases, you can retrain yourself to function without the self-conscious embarrassment you felt when you were young.

One of the goals of rehabilitation is to help you control bladder activity because it is one of the most important steps to independent living.

But there's more than the independence factor. There's the very real risk of infection, loss of pelvic muscle tone, and possible kidney problems if your bladder is not kept in check.

An important element of bladder training is fluid balance, which doesn't mean equal time for drinking and elimination. You need to take in more fluids than you put out in urine. Why? Bodily functions, such as sweating and even breathing, use some of the fluids you drink. If you don't take in *more* than you eventually release, you may end up dehydrated, which can be as dangerous to your health as too full a bladder.

The key is to maintain the right amounts of fluid at the right time; it helps your bladder management program by helping you know when it's time to go. Drink between 8 and 10 glasses of liquid a day, but try to avoid diuretic-like liquids, such as coffee, tea, colas, and alcohol. Avoid drinking fluids after dinner to reduce your nighttime trips to the bathroom. As part of your routine try to go to the bathroom every 2 to 4 hours, even if you don't feel the urge. This is called a timed voiding program.

If you aren't at your MS Rehabilitation Center every day, your team may ask you to keep your own "urine diary," using I & O for intake and output, at home—recording the times you go to the bathroom, as well as the amounts and types of fluids you drink. You'll also make scheduled "bathroom trips", trying different times, sometimes every half-hour, sometimes waiting an hour or two, sometimes 45 minutes. Eventually, you will become aware of when you need to void.

By regulating the amount of fluids you drink and by going to the bathroom at specific times each day, you help your body "learn" to eliminate at the appropriate time. *(Retraining also works for constipation and other stool problems. See the next section on bowel dysfunction.)*

A HEALTHY DOSE OF MEDICINE

There are drugs that can help control your bladder problems; they are most successful in treating incontinence and a spastic bladder. Some control the muscle (called the detrusor muscle) that contracts during urination; they help relieve spasms and the need to continually "go" by decreasing the amount of nerve transmissions that tell the bladder to empty. They give you much-needed time to get to a bathroom by lengthening the amount of time between each urge. These include tolterodine tartrate (Detrol®), oxybutynin (Ditropan®), hyoscyamine (Levsinex®, Levid®, and Cystospaz®), flavoxate hydrocholorid (Urispas®), propantheline bromide (Probanthine®), and imipramine (Tofranil®). Ditropan® is now supplied in a timed-release once-a-day pill. Called Ditropan XL®, it gives you a steady dose of oxybutynin all day long.

A flaccid bladder is easily managed by intermittent catheterization *(see the catheter section in this chapter)* to empty their bladder.

There has been success in treating detrusor sphincter dysynergia with alpha-adrenergic blockers (alpha blockers). Studies have found that they help improve bladder coordination and increase your control. These alpha-blockers include tamsulosin (Flomax®), phenoxybenzamine (Dibenzyline®), clonidine, and terazosin (Hytrin®). Dysynergia is best treated with a combination of medicines and a bladder diary.

Medicine is also given to relax the bladder and stop incontinent leaking—but intermittent catherization is still necessary to empty the stored urine. Remember, the goal is to stay dry and empty the bladder completely.

Your doctor will take into account your lifestyle, family history, and the severity of your problem to determine which method will work best for you.

WOMAN, YOUR NAME IS NOT VANITY

Injectable agents such as the collagen used by plastic surgeons to plump up wrinkles can now be injected directly into a woman's urinary sphincter. The collagen bulks up the sphincter, improving bladder control.

FEEL THE BURN: PELVIC EXERCISES

The pelvic floor muscles support and help control contractions in the bladder and the urethra. If you can strengthen these muscles, you can also better control your elimination flow. Pelvic floor muscles remind the brain to pay attention "down there." Some of the exercises used are:

Kegel. No, this is not the name of a new ethnic pastry. Kegel is an exercise designed specifically for women to help strengthen their pelvic floor and control their incontinence. The Kegel exercises are a study in control. While a woman is urinating, she should slowly "push in" or contract her pelvis. This stops the flow of urine. She should hold for 10 seconds, then release. The whole exercise should be repeated five or six times. Small, cone-shaped vaginal weights, in various degrees of heaviness, or devices called pessaries, can be inserted in a woman's vagina for extra strengthening before doing the exercise. The Kegel can be done at any time—at the gym, while a person is sitting and watching television, while she's still in bed, while she's washing her face, or even standing at the supermarket checkout line. The more a woman does the Kegel, the more she'll be able to control her elimination. (Please note: these exercises also work for men!)

The Valsalva maneuver. It might not look pretty, but this exercise can improve bladder emptying and decrease the risk of infection for weak bladder conditions. To do the Valsalva, you should be sitting on the toilet. Hold your breath, push down, trying to use your abdominal muscles, as if you were going to move your bowels. Then relax. Continue this maneuver until your bladder has emptied. Try double voiding for proper elimination: When you think you are done urinating, wait a minute, and then try voiding again. It will help get out the last bit of urine to help prevent infections.

(Although still in the research stage, valvular devices, which are inserted into a woman's urethra, open 8 to 10 seconds after the Valsalva is performed—and stay open for 3 minutes to ensure that the bladder is empty. These devices need to be changed every 3 months.)

A WARNING LABEL

The once popular Credé maneuver involves a pattern of kneading your fingers over your lower abdomen, then relaxing, over and over again until you have completely voided. Unfortunately, this is not safe for everyone. It can push urine up instead of down—and can damage your urinary tract and kidneys. Check with your doctor before trying this maneuver.

PERSONAL HYGENIE 101

The most common complication that can occur from bladder problems is a urinary tract infection (UTI)—which, untreated, can lead to kidney trouble. The symptoms of a UTI are similar to those of bladder dysfunction:

- A burning sensation when you urinate
- An urgent need to urinate, even after you've voided
- Frequent urination
- Blood in your urine
- Foul-smelling urine

It's important to see your doctor if you have any of these symptoms. He will do a urine culture test to see if your problem is a UTI or symptomatic of your bladder problems. A UTI is usually treated easily with antibiotics, but if you have frequent infections you will need to re-evaluate and change your routine.

You can also help avoid a UTI by wiping from front to back if you are a woman, drinking fluids to flush your system, avoiding delay in going to the bathroom, and drinking a daily glass of cranberry juice. Cranberries make the walls of the bladder and urethra too "slippery" for bacteria to cling to and grow.

If you have bladder problems, one of the most important things you can do to prevent infection doesn't take a great deal of time. It doesn't cost a lot of money. And it doesn't involve taking a pill. It's the motto of the nurse who taught health in school; one of the first rules of etiquette your parents told you: Wash your hands. That's it. If you remember to wash your hands after elimination, before and after using your catheter, you can drastically reduce your risk of infection. Take a cue from the surgeons in the OR: Wash up.

THE SECOND HALF OF THE STORY:
BOWEL DYSFUNCTION AND CONSTIPATION

Elimination is more than keeping an I & O sheet and a urine schedule. As we all know, the other normal human elimination function involves the bowel—and a different bodily system.

The gastrointestinal tract runs the whole length of the body. When you eat that pear or chocolate bar, saliva in the mouth begins to break it down and soften it for its journey down the gut. The food passes through the esophagus, the entrance to the stomach, and into the stomach itself. There, digestive action begins in earnest as that food is hit with stomach juices. Your pear, a complex carbohydrate, starts to break down into sugar (the good kind your body needs for fuel). Your candy bar becomes fat, sugar (the non-nutritive kind your body doesn't need), and a dollop of protein. Slowly

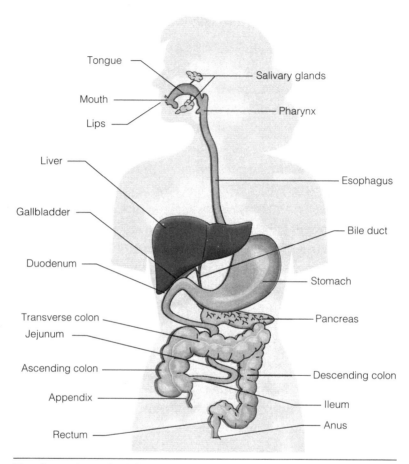

The Gastrointestinal System

this unrecognizable food travels to the small intestine where most of your digestive work takes place.

Here, in the small intestine, the food gets broken down even more, thanks to digestive juices, enzymes, and liver bile. The nutrients in the now unrecognizable pear or candy bar can then be sent to all parts of your body so hungry cells can eat (except for the chocolate bar's fat—which goes to those ubiquitous fat cells for storage).

WASTE-ING AWAY

Not every food you eat is used by the body. Where does it go? Liquid waste, as we have detailed in the previous section, eventually goes to the urinary tract. Bulk waste, on the other hand, goes from the small intestine into the large intestine, or colon. It is stored there, achieving bulk with undigested fiber and other by-products, until it gets its "cue" from the brain to leave the end of the large intestine, through the rectum, and out the anal sphincter muscles as stool.

In a perfect world, this process, like urination, is done without much thought. People develop routines; they have urges.

But when people develop MS, lesions and damaged myelin can develop at the base of the spinal cord (or in its nerve passageways that lead to the brain). The "fullness" cue may not get through to the anal sphincters passageways—or never even make it to the brain in the first place.

The result? Constipation, one of the most common symptoms in MS—and in life!

But, in addition to damaged myelin and short-circuited nerve passageways, there are other reasons why people with MS become constipated. These "Stubborn Stool Situations" include:

Stubborn Stool Situation #1: Weakness and Fatigue

Exercise is crucial for regularity. But when you have MS, it might not be possible to get the kind of exercise you need to keep pushing food through your intestines, turning it to waste, and keeping your bowels "on the move." When you feel weak and have trouble walking, it's possible that waste material begins to move much too slowly through the colon. Weak abdominal muscles can exacerbate the situation.

Stubborn Stool Situation #2: Spasticity

Spasticity doesn't just occur in your hands, arms, or legs. It can also occur in the muscles of your pelvic floor. If these muscles are unable to relax, you won't be able to have a normal bowel movement—and you'll become constipated.

Stubborn Stool Situation #3: Medication

It's a fact of life: People with MS have to take more medicine than most people—some of it preventative, some of it necessary to treat certain MS symptoms. Antidepressants. Calcium supplements. High blood pressure medicines. Antacids. Antihistamines. Pain medicines. One of the side effects of these drugs can be constipation. Make sure your doctor knows all the medications you are taking; he will know if one or more of them is causing constipation.

Stubborn Stool Situation #4: Lack of Fluids

The American Dietetic Association recommends drinking six to eight glasses of water a day, but most of us don't even come close. Caffeinated beverages, such as soda, coffee, and tea can soak up the extra liquids that we do consume. The result is dehydration—which leads to constipation. Add MS and the problem could become even more serious.

Some people with MS who have bladder problems will try to avoid embarrassment and discomfort by reducing the amount of liquid they drink. Not only can this cause dehydration, but you can also become constipated. And constipation can ultimately lead to so much stool build-up in the rectum that pressure is put on the urinary tract—causing the bladder problems you were trying to avoid.

SWALLOW THAT!

A nutritional assessment is crucial when getting a rehabilitation evaluation. Malnutrition, obesity, constipation, and problems swallowing (dysphagia) can all cause fatigue.

- *A serum albumin blood test can help see if you are suffering from malnutrition. A modified barium swallow (MBS) can help your doctor look at your swallowing mechanism.*
- *If your fatigue and accompanying weakness are caused by malnutrition, your doctor may prescribe a liquid supplement. If you don't like the taste, you can chill the can, then mix the contents with ice cream.*
- *If your appetite is gone and the lack of food is making you weak, your doctor may prescribe an appetite stimulant such as Megace®.*
- *If you are constipated, you will need to add fiber to your diet.*
- *If you cannot swallow, then you cannot drink or eat—which not only makes you weak, but terribly dependent on other people. The entire rehabilitation team, including your physician, speech pathologist, physical therapist, occupational therapist, nurse, dietitian—even a respiratory therapist and radiologist—will all help teach you to use weakened or tight throat muscles. Some strategies they may use include cutting pieces of food into small bits, chewing food thoroughly, eating slowly and pausing between swallows, and eating foods with a texture and consistency that are easier to swallow.*
- *And losing weight? We all know the answer to that one: Eat a healthy low-fat diet and do your prescribed exercises.*

Still, drinking fewer liquids is so common a behavior that many MS centers treat bladder problems *first* to ensure that a person is getting enough fluids for proper bowel function.

Unfortunately, constipation is an embarrassing topic. Like sex, it's a subject that many people feel uncomfortable talking about—including doctors! But bowel problems are very much a nuisance.

Constipation can keep you up at night—and worsen your fatigue during the day. It can make your spasticity worse, decrease your ability to walk, and, even worse, create incontinence.

Ironically, constipation is one of the easiest symptoms of MS to treat. It just takes some time, patience, and the confidence to discuss it with a member of your rehabilitation team.

CREATING A BOWEL PROGRAM

The first step to regularity is planning. As with bladder dysfunction, timing is everything. Set up a bowel movement schedule based on the time of day that is most convenient for you. Although work, family commitments, or travel can get in the way, the ideal time to head to the toilet is 15 to 30 minutes after you've eaten; there will be more movement in the bowel. Try to keep to this schedule even if you don't feel the urge. If it seems to be taking a longer time to move your bowels, try sipping some warm coffee, tea, or water; they help stimulate peristalsis (the movement of stools through the large intestine). You can also try digitally manipulating the sphincter muscle. (Always wear plastic gloves to avoid infection.)

DON'T UNDERSTIMATE A HEALTHY DIET

A fiber-rich diet. It's a phrase you've heard over and over again in books, in the news, in magazines. But it's not hype. A fiber-rich diet is healthy for you. Fiber is not digested.

Instead this plant material holds water. What does this mean to your bowels? Easy. It helps keep your stool moving down your colon by adding bulk to the stool waste and, at the same time, softening it with water. Fiber not only helps constipation, it helps prevent gas, bloating, and even diarrhea!

You'll find fiber in fruits, vegetables, nuts, seeds, and whole grains. If you haven't made fiber a habit, your best bet is to start slowly. Too much fiber all at once can cause havoc in your digestive system, creating gas and bloating. Gradually adding fiber to your diet every day can help avoid this "shock" to your system.

Make sure you also drink your water (in accordance with your bladder program)! Liquids help facilitate fiber's "magic."

If you cannot tolerate the side effects of fiber, all is not lost. You can also add fiber to your diet via a supplement. If your mobility is limited, you'll also need more fiber than you can get from diet alone. Some supplements work better than others for different people. Experiment. Supplements include bran, psyllium hydrophilic muciloid (Metamucil®, FiberCon®, Citrucel®), and calcium polycarbophil.

ONE, TWO, THREE, REPEAT . . . EXERCISE

Regular physical activity also helps stimulate peristalsis. It helps keep stool moving through your colon—not to mention the good work it does for your cardiovascular system. In short, exercise is crucial for regularity. If you are a sedentary person, your elimination system is not going to work efficiently. Taking a walk in loose, cool clothing (to that point *before* fatigue sets in!), swimming, or—if you use a wheelchair or

THE OPPOSITE SIDE OF THE COIN: DIARRHEA

Although much less common than constipation, diarrhea and its consequences can be much more severe for people with MS: it can cause incontinence. When you experience a loss of sensation in the rectal area (caused by myelin damage to the nerve passageways in the spinal cord), the rectum may stretch too much and trigger the anal sphincter muscles to relax—releasing watery, loose stool. Medications such as Pro-Banthine® or Ditropan® can help, as can bulk-forming supplements such as Metamucil®.
(When a bulk-forming medicine is used for diarrhea, instead of constipation, do not drink any water with it—but don't avoid liquids during the day. You want to firm the stool—but not cause constipation.)

And remember, diarrhea can be caused by problems other than your MS. See your doctor to rule out any gastrointestinal illnesses.

scooter—range-of-motion exercises and upper-arm stretches can all help keep your bowels on a smooth, regular course.

WHEN ALL ELSE FAILS: MEDICINE THAT WORKS

Sometimes man and woman cannot live on healthy habits alone. Perhaps you do your aqua aerobics faithfully three times a week. Maybe you are religious about getting to the bathroom at the same time every day. And maybe you take your fiber supplement and eat lots of fruits and vegetables—all to no avail.

There is still hope. Good medicines are out there and they can help. These include:

Stool softeners. If your constipation is caused by consistently hard stool, softeners such as Colace® or Surfax®, which are taken morning and night, or Chronulac® syrup, starting with 1 ounce in the evening, can help.

Mild laxatives. These oral stimulants help promote water secretion into the colon—which irritates it, forcing a "smoother move." Laxatives are used if your trouble is pushing the stool out. Because laxatives can be habit-forming (you won't be able to move your bowels without them!), do not take harsh ones such as the over-the-counter chocolate-flavored tablets. Mild laxatives, or oral stimulants, do the job just as well in about 8 to 12 hours. The best ones to use include Pericolace® (which is the stool softener Colace® with an added stimulant) and Milk of Magnesia®. Follow the directions on the bottle.

Suppositories and Enemas. If your constipation does not respond to any of these medications or nutritional changes, you might need a more powerful stimulant. Suppositories and enemas provide both a chemical irritant and sphincter muscle stimulation. They include:

√ *Glycerin suppositories.* These do not contain any medicine, but they do offer rectal stimulation and lubrication. Because they are fairly mild, suppositories can be very useful when you are first establishing your bowel program.

√ *Dulcolax® suppositories* do contain medicine—and are, consequently, stronger. They work by stimulating a wavelike motion in the muscles of the rectum.

√ *Therevac® mini-enemas.* These come in wrapped "shells" that conveniently and cleanly lubricate the rectal muscles.

√ *Enemas* must be used sparingly. Like harsh laxatives, they can become habit-forming and should be used only infrequently. Fleet® is an enema used in many diagnostic tests to "clean out" the colon.

This ends our journey through the MS symptoms landscape. But there is still more to come: the ride home.

PART FOUR

THE RIDE HOME

CHAPTER FOURTEEN

THE ACTIVITIES
OF DAILY LIVING

I thought I'd be doomed to always asking someone,
my husband, my therapist, my daughter, to help me
cook a meal. I just couldn't reach up to get the ingre-
dients I needed; I couldn't cut food. When I had an
acute attack, I couldn't even feed myself. That was
truly horrible. But thanks to my MS support group, I
learned about devices I could buy to help me be inde-
pendent, knives, forks, even extenders. For the first
time in a very long time I felt free!

—A 53-year-old female professor
with Secondary-Progressive MS

- It had taken a while, but Todd finally learned how to get dressed by himself. But he never quite mastered putting on his shoes and socks. His MS had made his fingers clumsy, and he had difficulty bending down and tying a shoe at the same time. His fingers refused to work in unison. Does this mean he has to live the rest of his life barefoot—or dependent on someone else? No! The solution: a long-handled shoehorn, a special adaptive device for putting on socks, and loafers instead of the oxfords he'd always worn.
- Mary Beth had been left with some cognitive problems after her last MS attack. She could remember things about her past, music she liked, even the names of the people she loved. But she had trouble with recent memory and more complex tasks. When she wanted to

255

pay her bills, she couldn't always remember to do it on time. When she took a shower, she couldn't remember if she had used soap. When it was her turn to host her bridge group, she would forget until everyone appeared at her door. The solution? An individual "how-to" book designed specifically for her, spelling out, step-by-step, the various tasks, including when and how to do them.

- Ellen loved to take baths but she was sure that after her last MS attack, they would be a thing of the past. She had trouble walking; she couldn't balance her body; she needed a scooter quite a few hours out of the day. There was no way she could get herself into a tub without falling. Besides, she had a sensitivity to heat. But that was before a local handyman came to her house and put up grab bars, steps, and a special control on the faucet that would prevent the water from getting too hot.

Independence is achieved from the simple, ordinary routines that we take for granted. As these examples show, adapting to a disability or relearning the activities of daily living (ADLs) can make all the difference between leading a life dependent on others—or living free, independent, and self-reliant.

Because ADLs are so important, rehabilitation teams, especially occupational therapists, spend a great deal of time and energy on them. There are also special catalogues where you can order adaptive equipment to help you design an environment that helps keep you as independent as possible.

LIFE IS COMPLICATED

Getting dressed. Using the toilet. Brushing your teeth and bathing. These may seem like minor things, ordinary, simple actions that shouldn't be too difficult to relearn. They shouldn't require a whole lot of attention. Wrong! Take a look at the steps required to take an early morning shower.

1. Take off pajamas and hang them on a hook.
2. Turn on the water.
3. Regulate the temperature.
4. Step into the tub or stall.
5. Wet body and hair.
6. Open shampoo bottle and pour some in hands.
7. Wash hair.
8. Rinse.
9. Pick up soap in dish.
10. Soap up body, including toes and underarms.
11. Pick up washcloth.
12. Scrub behind the ears and work up a lather all over.
13. Put down washcloth.
14. Wash off soap well.
15. Turn off water.
16. Get out of tub or stall.
17. Reach for towel.
18. Dry hair and body.

This simple, everyday task required 18 steps alone—and that didn't even take putting on body lotion, deodorant, and undergarments into account.

Here's another one: brushing your teeth. It's an easy routine for someone who has full use of her arms and hands to open a tube of toothpaste and turn on the water. But what if someone couldn't hold a regular thin toothbrush? What if, at times, she was too weak to squeeze the tube? And what if she had difficulty finding the toothpaste or the brush? Suddenly, a very routine act becomes complicated.

Let's go over the functions brushing your teeth utilizes so you can see exactly how intricate ADLs are:

1. *Visual:* You need to see your toothbrush, toothpaste, and rinsing cup, not to mention the sink.
2. *Cognitive.* You have to remember that it's morning and you should brush your teeth.
3. *Motor.* You have to use your arm, hands, and fingers to get that brush going—not to mention opening the tube of toothpaste.
4. *Sensory.* You have to feel the texture of the brush against your teeth and the handle in your hand. Are you brushing too hard? Too soft?
5. *Perceptual.* Exactly how far do you have to move your arm to reach your mouth? How far back inside your mouth do you go?
6. *Coordination.* Putting toothpaste on the brush. Bringing the brush up to your mouth. Rinsing with water and spitting it out. All these steps require the coordination of your eyes and your mouth, your arms and your hands.

Most people with MS remember how to do these simple tasks. (Remember, only 10% have severe cognitive difficulties.) But many people with MS will have difficulty *performing* them. They have to find ways to compensate for their disabilities. Here are some suggestions to make life easier— from the home to the office, from eating to watching TV, from traveling to going out.

HOME, AGAIN

When you first moved into your house or apartment, you designed it according to your taste—the colors you like, the furniture you find comfortable, the rugs, drapes, and pictures that match your style.

When your symptoms of MS begin to affect your ability to get around, you may have to modify your home. Think of it as a design problem—not as a plan for a sterile hospital room. Home is where you can put your feet up, and more than any other place, you need to make it accessible, safe, and comfortable. The more your house is designed around you, the less energy you will expend on daily routines—and the less you will feel fatigued.

There's even a name for making your house disability-friendly: It's called accessibility and it is, quite simply, a way to a better quality of life at home. This isn't as complicated as it sounds; you will rarely need a "rehabilitation engineering specialist" to help design your home to conform to your needs. Your therapists, rehabilitation hospital, and the Internet are all excellent resources. Ramps, grab bars, bathroom fixtures, extra door widths, wider entryways, lighting—these are all part of a day's work for rehabilitation professionals. They will suggest modified environmental controls, such as special light switches, heat and air controls, and alarm systems, to help you maintain independence in your house—and your workplace, too. (Your therapist, doctor, or the National Multiple Sclerosis Society at 1-800-FIGHT MS will be able to provide you with the names of resources in your area. They can also provide helpful suggestions for you to "do-it-yourself".) A case manager, who works with people with disabilities, knows where to obtain all of these items at the best price and can act as your rehabilitation "contractor."

Things that went unnoticed before you developed MS are now under scrutiny. How do you get into your house? How do you get up the stairs? How do you get enough light for you to see well enough to read? How do you open the kitchen cupboards with weakened hands? The medicine cabinet? How do you go from room to room? How do you get out fast in case of fire? How can you answer a door or telephone when walking across the foyer is no longer easy?

A doorway may need to be wide enough for you to turn around in while using your mobility aids or sitting on a scooter. You may need your sink lowered to a workable level along with extra free space under your counter tops. You might need a doorway that is at least 32 inches and preferably 36 inches wide to accommodate your wheelchair. You might need a door with a lever latch that opens easily with one motion. You might need cabinets that open easily, drawers that you can close, closets where you can hang all your clothes within reach on a lower rod.

Some hints to ensure your home is comfortable, accessible, and safe:

Hearth and Home

- If you don't need your upstairs floors, don't use them. Make sure you arrange your ground floor with everything you may need.
- If you use a scooter or wheelchair, remember that your easy-reach zone starts at approximately 15-16 inches from the floor and ends at 51-52 inches. When you stand, the zone starts at your knees and ends just a few inches higher than your head—*not your outstretched arms.*
- Forget about doorsills! They can bump and hit and catch you unawares. Have all doorsills between rooms

removed. If getting rid of a doorsill is impossible, there is still good news: Companies that specialize in adaptive equipment sell small ramps that can help you move from room to room.

- Keep ramps no steeper than one foot of length for each inch of height. In other words, a six-foot long ramp should only rise six inches.
- Add protective shields or insulation to any exposed pipes and motors. You don't want to be surprised by a burn or scrape!
- Make sure you have at least two emergency exits in your home. Common sense for all of us.
- Think "outdoors" for doors. They should never swing in as they can bump into you and cause injuries.
- Keep an alarm system nearby—a keypad, if possible, that links you to the fire department and the police with a simple light touch of a button. One that you can wear around your neck or keep in your purse is ideal. Don't respond to those TV ads that show a person on the floor—they are very expensive. Most local hospitals offer this service at a much lower cost.
- Fire drills really do have a purpose—in today's secure-conscious world more than ever. Have fire drills in your own home, with your family, so they will not only know how to get out of the house safely—but can help you reach safety as well. This is especially important if you use a wheelchair or any assistive devices.

Lighting Up Your Life

- Traditional on-off light switches can be replaced with user-friendly rocker panels that enable people with weakness to use their arms, elbows, or palms of their

hands to bring light into a room. A light switch exten-
der, found in hardware stores or specialty catalogues,
can lower the actual switch up to 15 inches for easier
accessibility.

- Even discount stores now have lamps that are "touch-
sensitive." Instead of turning a light on or off with a
switch, you merely have to touch its base. Some of
these lamps run on batteries and you can easily place
several throughout the house.
- Dimmers are easy to install and are easier to use than
switches.
- If you are having difficulty with your vision, make sure
that mirrors and paintings are hung high and out of
your way. Keep your house free from clutter that could
be bumped into and cause injury.
- Cover or refinish shiny, reflective surfaces. They can
interfere with your ability to see.
- Clearly mark thermostats, stove controls, toaster
ovens, and any other dials that need to be read.
Bright red nail polish can immediately tell you when
something is off or on—or where the optimal temperature is.
- Paint the edges of steps and doorways in a contrasting
color from the walls. This will ensure that you won't
tumble if you are having trouble seeing as you walk
from room to room.

Telephone Calls

- There are many different types of devices that can
make using your telephone easier than ever. Hands-free
headsets are invaluable for both home phone use and

cell phones. In fact, in many states they're the law. They enable you to speak and listen without blocking out any important background noise.

- There are shoulder holders you can get for your phone. They allow the phone to sit on your shoulder without hurting your neck.
- If you have trouble seeing or have poor hand coordination, there are telephones with big numbers and large buttons for easy access. The same is true for TV remote control devices.
- Check with your phone company: There are many different types of service available for people who may have trouble with their vision, hearing, or range-of-motion. Voice-activated phones mean you don't even need to dial. Volume control devices can act like hearing aids, helping you adjust the sound of the rings as well as your conversations. Speed-dialing cuts down on the number of times you need to "punch" a button. (Keep a list of the numbers and names of people you speed-dial by the phone. Better yet, attach it to the phone table or the body of the phone so you don't misplace it. Many phones will store those frequently called numbers for you.)

Using the Bathroom

- Elevated toilet seats can ease the strain of sitting down and getting back up by raising the seat four to seven inches. You can even get them with armrests for added comfort. You can also go the handyman route and have a wall-mounted grab bar attached to your bathroom wall at the right level for you.

- There are products out there that can make showering a lot easier: A shower caddy or a hanging basket that fits over the shower head can hold all your shampoos, conditioners, and gel washes within easy reach.
- Make sure you use a non-skid mat on the tub or shower floor.
- Shower chairs can help if you are unsteady on your feet.
- Grab bars placed strategically on the tub or shower wall will help give you a "lift" when you want to get out or need assistance to maintain your balance.
- Need help moving your shower curtain back and forth? Try rubbing some Vaseline® on your shower curtain rod.
- Keep your medicine cabinet neat and orderly; it will help you find things fast without tiring your arms. Small magnets inside the front door can hold cuticle scissors, mustache clippers, nail files—anything metal that you might need.
- A plain old spice rack can "second" as a great medicine bottle holder—that's clearly seen at eye level.
- Throw out that old makeup and those dusty free samples. Instead, use one of your bathroom drawers to store clean underwear. You'll be able to go from the shower to getting dressed in one room.
- Telescoping mirrors can help if your medicine cabinet mirror is too high for you to see yourself. Many also come with lights and a magnifying feature.
- If your hands are weak, use bath mittens or a soft "scrunchy" to wash yourself instead of a harder-to-hold washcloth.

Kitchen Helpers

- Remove the doors from your kitchen cabinets. It's so much easier to find something if you don't have to deal with a door that may stick.
- If you find that the kitchen countertops are either too high or have insufficient space underneath to accommodate your scooter or wheelchair, you might need to have a carpenter come in and modify them. If it's not possible to do a revamp of your whole kitchen, check out the costs of just adding one or two lower sections that you can use more easily.
- Gather everything together that you'll need to make a meal. This way you can sit down and prepare it—without getting up and down.
- A sticky product called Dycem™ can hold pots in place while you stir them; you can find it in health food stores.
- Businesses give them away the same way they give out magnets. They're those round rubbery sheets that "hug" a jar and make it easier to open. You can also try using a rubber glove.
- Think easy: frozen, canned, pre-packaged meals, take out—these are the easiest to cook and clean up after.
- Take advantage of aluminum foil. Use it to line baking pans, grills, whatever will take the grease. Even better, use disposable aluminum pans that you can buy in the supermarket. Either way, clean-up's a breeze.
- The microwave is your friend. Just make sure it's perched at a level that's comfortable for you to reach when sitting down.
- Don't be shy about asking for help.
- Slide heavy items across counter tops instead of picking them up.

- If you have trouble reaching your sink, think rubber tub. But instead of filling the tub with soapy water, invert it—so that the bottom is up. Voila! An instant platform that can be reached more easily for washing dishes and cleaning up.
- Do what restaurants do: When emptying the dishwasher, set the table for the next meal. That's one less chore you'll have to do before you eat!

In the Bedroom

- Make your bed without walking around its entire perimeter by making up one side completely before going to the other side. A two-foot dowel with a hook at the end can help you smooth out blankets and bedspreads.
- Everyone wants to feel warm and cozy at night—but not weighed down by blankets. Choose warm but lightweight blankets that don't add any additional discomfort.
- Move your bed against one wall if you have trouble turning in your sleep. Add a grab bar at a height that's comfortable for you, and you'll be able to turn around whenever you are in bed.
- Keep a flashlight on the night table! You never know when you'll need it. It's also easier to grab a flashlight than to turn on the light. Just make sure they are lightweight and have an easy-to-use on/off switch.
- Keep your closets user-friendly by ensuring that shelves and clothes rods are low enough for you to reach without straining. Avoid time-consuming (and sometimes painful) searching by labeling shoeboxes and keeping shirts and sweaters separate with plastic bins.

I CAN DO THIS!

It's one thing to ensure your house is safe and accessible, to know that you can reach shelves, climb into bathtubs, and turn the lights off in a room without asking for help. But the greatest accomplishments come from doing things yourself. Whether it be as basic as getting dressed or as complex as using your computer at work, performing your routine chores and rituals will create confidence and personal empowerment.

Here are some suggestions to get you moving—independently:

Getting Dressed

- Remember: Velcro is easier to deal with than buttons and zippers.
- Keep clothes loose and comfortable with as little fastening needed as possible. A hint: Shop at a maternity store. The clothes will be loose—and fashionable, too!
- Cotton might feel good, but 100% cotton will shrink and show every wrinkle. Instead, opt for the new Tencel® blends or a combination of cotton and polyester.
- Keep accessories simple. Instead of a hat and scarf in cold weather, wear an all-in-one. Purchase a raincoat with an attached hood. It can act as a great umbrella.
- Clip-on earrings are easier to maneuver than pierced ones.
- Simple, solid colors will not camouflage buttons and buttonholes—unlike bright plaids or complicated designs. This is especially important if you are having difficulties with your vision.

- Belts should be woven through the loops *before* donning pants.
- Front-fastening bras are easier to put on.
- Getting a shirt or blouse on is easier if you are sitting down with your feet flat on the floor. Put the shirt on your lap, then lean over. This way you'll be able to use your good arm to push a weakened or spastic arm through its sleeve. Follow the collar around your neck with your good hand, then push that same hand through the remaining sleeve.
- This same process works for putting on pants, but with one difference. Cross a weakened or spastic leg over the stronger leg; the stronger arm helps push up the slacks leg. Once the pant leg is on, the legs can be uncrossed, and the procedure can be followed again with the stronger leg (and arm).
- Button shirts from bottom to top to ensure proper alignment.
- Use your adaptive equipment! There are a myriad of devices out there that can help you dress by yourself. These include buttonhooks, extra-long shoehorns, and snaps instead of buttons.
- A golden rule: What is put on first, comes off last.

Eating a meal

- Think light—and not just when you are eating a meal. We've already gone over the reasons why a low-fat, fiber-rich diet *(see Chapter 13)* can keep you strong. But light can also pertain to dishes. Frankly, plastic dishes are easier and more flexible to use than china. If you'd rather use "real" dishware, opt for Melamine™ or Corelle™; both are lighter than regular dishes.

- When eating pizza, don't reach for that unwieldy triangle. Instead, cut the pizza up into smaller pieces; it will be easier to maneuver and chew.
- Dishes that contrast with the tabletop will make it easier to see when eating.
- Forget about sugar bowls—or any other serving piece that can possibly fall and create a mess. Instead, fill clean salt shakers up with your sugar or artificial sweetener.
- Napkins might be a part of proper etiquette, but when dining at home, use a towel. It's more absorbent, and bits of food won't spill out into your lap.
- If you have problems grasping and holding onto silverware, you can use modeling clay to build up the handle. You can also purchase special adapative equipment that can help you cut food as well as take the place of knives and forks.
- Salad forks are lighter than regular forks.
- Serrated knives make cutting meat easier.
- You're not being a baby if you use baby warming plates. If you eat more slowly, they'll prevent your food from getting cold.
- Thermal mugs are not just for cars. They'll keep your beverage hot or cold and, as an added plus, they're easier to grasp.
- Use a pie plate with a rim if you have problems with food sliding off your dish. Similarly, if your dish slides around on the table, the same plastic suction cups used in showers to hold washcloths or sponges will hold it in place.
- Elevating a plate can also help. Trays with legs, a sturdy box, or specially designed "lifts" that you can find in a medical equipment catalogue can all do the trick.

**YOU DON'T HAVE TO DO IT ALONE
—OR WITH PAIN**

*Adaptive equipment can really make a difference—
but, unfortunately, many people with MS don't know
it exists! One of the best catalogues around is from
the AbilityOne Corporation. It contains everything
from exercise "putty" to increase hand strength to
rocker knifes, long-handled brushes to reachers. (You
can find its address and phone number in the appendix at the back of this book.)*

Personal hygiene and you

- Shower or bathe in cool water to keep your body temperature down. But, ouch!, don't start with cold water
  right away. Rather, begin your showering with tepid
  water, gradually making it cooler as you get used to it.
- Cotton dishcloths will work better than terry washcloths if your hands are weak.
- Purchase long-handled combs and brushes.
- Cut your toenails *after* your shower. They'll be nice and
  soft and easier to cut.
- Dental floss now comes in all different shapes and
  sizes. The best one for someone with MS symptoms is
  the one that has a sturdy plastic handle and a "line" of
  floss attached to each of its ends like a tiny clothesline.
  These disposable flosses come in packages with a full
  month's supply.

- Electric toothbrushes and Water Piks promote independence in dental hygiene.
- Electric shavers are better than razor blades, for obvious reasons.
- Spray deodorants are easier to use with one hand.
- Think glamour: Purchase a vanity dresser or create a makeshift one with a table, a chair, and a mirror. Put your makeup, tweezers, and cotton swabs in drawers that are at the right height for you—as well as the position of the mirror. You'll be able to put on everything from eyeliner to blush easily and correctly.

These are only a few examples of how Activities of Daily Living can be performed—despite your MS symptoms. Your occupational therapist will help you in your routines. Don't be afraid to ask questions.

There's still one area we have yet to "visit", one stop on our journey we still have to make. It's alternative therapy—the natural way that some people use to treat multiple sclerosis. Does it work? You'll find out next. . . .

CHAPTER FIFTEEN

ALTERNATIVE THERAPY: DOES IT WORK?

There's only one bottom line for me: I'll try anything
to reduce my multiple sclerosis symptoms. I don't
care if it's an herb, a magnet, or a new medical drug.

—A 38-year-old female management consultant
with relapsing-remitting MS

Close your eyes and imagine yourself back in time, to the days when humans lived in caves and their daily routine was all about survival. When someone got sick, it was considered fate, an angry god seeking revenge. In a dark cave, lit by flickering flames from a nearby fire, a shaman might perform rituals to stave off death. He would dance and chant and throw herbs and seeds into the fire. Sparks would fly; his painted face illuminated in the brief burst of light. But this medicine, despite the authority of the shaman, was more about luck than knowledge. More times than not, the sick person was left to die as the tribe migrated on its journey for food. Only the strong and the healthy lived another day.

Now travel in warp time to the ancient golden cultures — to Egypt, Greece, and Rome. Here, in these advanced cultures, doctors were revered and anatomy and physiology studied intensely. They understood the importance of cleanliness even if they didn't understand the concept of germs. The sick were treated and the dead studied for clues. Although these physicians knew nothing about modern drugs and diagnostic scans, they knew about the properties found in herbs, plants, flowers, and seeds. Along with their rituals and prayers, these doctors used nature to cure the sick—and it sometimes worked. Certain herbs are natural antibiotics. Certain flowers, tree barks, and seeds could effectively treat heart ailments, arthritis, infection, pulmonary problems, and flu.

Even when these golden cultures fell and the Dark Ages spread across Western Europe, this knowledge of herbs and plants did not die. Now it was the women who passed on their information from healer to healer. Although they were sometimes burned at the stake for being witches, these healers played an important role in helping the sick get well.

But healers were no match against epidemics, against the plague or smallpox. Only modern medicine, a burgeoning discipline, would be able to stop them in their tracks.

Over time those "old-fashioned" natural cures were pushed aside as medicine performed its miracles. Suddenly there were pills that could fight infection, injections that could prevent illness, diagnostic tools that could determine what the problem was—and where. Science and research continued to grow throughout the 20th and into the 21st century, delving into molecular biology, probing areas of the brain never before dissected, and learning about specific diseases, predispositions, and root causes of illness that would have rendered our ancestors speechless.

Today, however, natural medicine (also called complementary and alternative medicine, or CAM) has had a comeback. The expense of various medicines, the side-effects of these medicines, and the trend among people today for natural, organic things—all these have played a part in the emergence once again of alternative medicine.

But, above all, alternative medicine has gained popularity because it provides new hope. When traditional, acceptable therapies don't work, when the side-effects are too disabling, when nothing seems to "cure" the disease—in these cases, alternative medicine is turned to, held on to, and fervently used to help find relief.

As in so many other serious situations, people with multiple sclerosis—a disabling disease that can affect a person during her entire adult life—turn to alternative medicines. After all, MS is a disease that seems to strike with no rhyme or reason. Alternative medicines not only offer hope to people with MS, but also offer the illusion of control over a disease that is cruelly unpredictable.

And, most importantly, doctors today are not opposed to many natural remedies: A healthy diet, routine exercise, yoga and meditation, sleep, vitamin and mineral supplements, and acupuncture are all "alternatives" that have been found to help decrease the symptoms of disease. Medicine alone is no longer king. Drug therapy can live side by side with alternative therapy.

The key is in knowing which natural therapies will complement traditional medicine—and which ones only provide false hope.

In this chapter, we will examine some of the more common alternative therapies currently being used by people to help reduce their multiple sclerosis symptoms. Together, we will see which ones are valid—and why.

But before we begin, let's first see what's true about alternative medicines—and what is possibly dangerous myth.

THE TRUTH PREVAILS

Alternative medicine has a huge following. And, as it's grown, certain ideas and beliefs have built up around it. They may be considered the truth by many people, but, in fact, they are completely false. Here are the common myths surrounding alternative medicine—and the realities that should take their place.

Myth #1: Alternative means natural—and natural means safe.

Wrong! Just because something is "natural," grown in the earth or processed only by nature, it doesn't mean that it is safe to use. Poison ivy is natural—and certainly toxic. Jack o'lantern mushrooms can kill you. Arsenic is a natural-occurring element formed in the earth—and it has killed more people throughout history than any other poison.

In short, just because something is natural doesn't mean it isn't toxic. There are dangers in nature just as there may be in certain drugs or combinations of drugs.

Myth #2: Why not try alternative medicine? What do you have to lose, except maybe time or money. There's no real health risks.

This myth is usually combined with the one above: Alternative medicine is, at worst, ineffectual. It can't make your condition *worse*, right? Wrong again. Risk is a part of life. Whether it's a diagnostic test in the hospital or a supplement taken with juice, taking action has some degree of risk. True, some procedures, medications, and alternative therapies have less risk than others—but less does not mean risk-free. The question you need to ask yourself before beginning *any* medical regimen is "Do the benefits outweigh the risks?" Talk to your doctor. Explore the Internet. Once you are armed with information, you can make the right decision for yourself.

Myth #3: Alternative medicine is pain free.

Guess again. Alternative medicines are not just the vitamins you swallow in the morning or the yoga you practice at night. Within this same category is colonic irrigation (involving powerful laxatives to "cleanse" your intestines), chelation therapy (in which an acid is injected into your body), and mercury filling removal (remember the last time you went to the dentist!) These procedures are all invasive. They can be painful—and potentially dangerous to your health. (*We'll be going over these therapies and others later in this chapter.*)

Myth #4: Finding an alternative therapy is like finding a rare jewel. You will be the miracle worker, the one who finds a miracle cure.

Sadly, there is no "blue Bombay diamond" tucked away on some link in the Internet. There is no extraordinary cure for MS. If there were, it wouldn't be hidden: everyone would be using it!

But people keep searching and keep believing that an alternative course will stave off their diseases, their infections, their old age. In fact, Americans spend more than $27 billion every year on alternative medicines.

This figure increases in people who have a chronic disease—like multiple sclerosis. Many studies have shown that at least three-fourths of people with MS have tried alternative medicines to help stave off the disease. And this number crosses all incomes, all genders, all education levels, and all ages.

But nothing is more telling than the findings of one particular Danish study: The use of alternative medicines declines as MS progresses and worsens.

Myth #5: Don't tell your doctor.
He'll never understand!

This myth only leads to trouble. It's imperative that you let your doctor "in" on your "secret." He should be informed of any vitamins, supplements, or alternative therapies you are using in conjunction with your conventional medicines. Why? Because only he can determine if these therapies are contraindicated, causing harm to you when combined with your regular medicines. Only he can tell you if there is a risk of toxicity involved in your treatments. Remember: Your doctor is your partner in your MS journey. He is not the enemy. If

---

ALTERNATIVE MEDICINE TURNS LEGIT

Once the sole province of health foods stores, obscure mail-order catalogues, and solitary wellness centers, alternative medicine has become mainstream. This new-found respect became official in 1992, when the U.S. National Institutes of Health created the Office of Alternative Medicine (OAM) to fund research that studies the safety and effectiveness of alternative medicine. Funding those institutions and laboratories researching CAMs would put alternative therapies under the same scientific scrutiny that traditional medicine undergoes as a matter of course. (Conventional medicine must be approved by the Food and Drug Administration before being marketed; alternative medicine does not . . . yet.) Unfortunately, results have been mixed—but long-term studies have yet to be analyzed.

he is a good doctor, he will be open to CAM (complementary/alternative medicine). These therapies can *complement* (not take the place of) your traditional medicine and help ease your symptoms—and your doctor should know that.

Myth #6: *If you improve while taking alternative medicine, it means it's working!*

Not necessarily. Of course, any improvement is a reason for cheering—and you should feel good if your symptoms subside. But that improvement may not be from your therapy. As we have already seen, multiple sclerosis is an uncharted disease; it is unpredictable, and you never know when a remission or remittance will occur. Your improvement could just be the natural course of your particular MS journey—and have nothing to do with the alternative medicine you are taking.

You could also be experiencing a placebo effect: This is a situation in which you want the medicine to work so much that you psychologically believe it has. (A placebo is a sugar pill that gets its name from scientific studies: half the subjects are given the "real thing" while an equal number get a placebo.) Research shows that many of the people who take only a placebo actually have positive results. This phenomenon is called "the placebo effect," and scientists must take it into account when they analyze their studies. A good study will compare the alternative medicine to a placebo in a "double blind" study where neither the patients nor the physician knows which ones are being taken until the study is over. This is the standard used in research studies on regular medicines, but it is rarely done with alternative therapies and medicines.

COMMON CAMS

In the world of complementary and alternative medicines, there are as many choices as there are in more traditional modes of therapy. To help you separate the wheat from the chaff, the real thing from the scam, we've included a brief collection of the most common CAMs people with multiple sclerosis have tried:

"Acid Trip": Chelation Therapy

What Is It? The word chelation literally means "the process of combining with and dissolving." In this case, a crystalline acid (EDTA) is intravenously injected over a period of several hours. As the acid moves through your bloodstream, it chelates (read: binds) any heavy metals it finds floating around. These theoretically toxic metals are then excreted out of your body via the kidneys.

How Effective Is It? Although chelation therapy is used for lead poisoning and rare disorders involving metal accumulation in the bloodstream, there is no proof that it works for any of the diseases it is touted to help: arthritis, strokes, Parkinson's disease—and MS. These conditions have nothing to do with the build-up of metal in the body.

How Expensive Is It? Very. The treatment requires several months—and up to $6000.

Any Dangers? Yes. *Chelation therapy has significant risks to your health.* It can cause kidney damage and can be lethal to certain individuals.

"Full Metal Jacket": Removal of Mercury Fillings

What Is It? Those silver and mercury amalgam fillings put in by your dentist are removed and replaced with a non-metal substance. Advocates of this therapy say that mercury leaks from the fillings can damage the immune system; the mercury is also said to leak into the root canal nerve and cause autoimmune problems.

How Effective Is It? It isn't. Studies show that people with multiple sclerosis have the same levels of mercury as other people. Although mercury poisoning can damage the nervous system and lead to tremors and weakness, the root cause of the nerve damage is completely different than it is for MS.

How Expensive Is It? Think about the last time you saw your dentist: Any kind of dental work does not come cheap.

Any Dangers? Removing old fillings can be painful and time consuming. Manipulating your teeth can also cause further dental problems, such as root canal nerve damage. (If you want caps or porcelain veneers to look better, that is one thing. But don't have your fillings removed because you think it will help your MS!)

"From Ancient Times": T'ai Chi

What Is It? T'ai Chi, an ancient Chinese regimen of meditative, repetitive exercises, has entered the mainstream gym and workout center. By concentrating on the same gentle movements, your body and mind are brought into balance.

How Effective Is It? This exercise, like yoga, is excellent for relaxation, stress reduction, and balance strengthening whether you are able-bodied or disabled. It can be performed by anyone, no matter your age or physical condition.

How Expensive Is It? T'ai Chi is relatively inexpensive. The only costs are the classes or a video.

Any Dangers? No. T'ai Chi exercises are completely safe. If you have difficulty with your mobility, you can even do them in a chair.

"The Sting" or Snake and Honey Bee Therapy
What Is It? Exactly what they sound like: stings. In theory, honey bee venom—from live honey bee stings—enters your bloodstream to stimulate your immune system. Apitherapy, its scientific name, is rich in the polyunsaturated fat that, supposedly, people with MS lack in sufficient amounts.

Snake bites are not part of the therapy in snake venom therapy—but the venom itself is. Called PROven, Venogen, or Horvi MS9, this venom is a mixture of cobra, krait, and water moccasin venoms; it is given by subcutaneous injection. The assumption is that the venom is rich in many of the proteins and enzymes that people with MS lack; it is purported to stimulate normal enzymatic function, strengthening the immune system and weakening any virus growth. Snake venom therapy is also believed to reduce inflammation and pain.

How Effective Is It? Unfortunately, studies have not born out any of these claims—for either honey bee venom or snake venom. The FDA has banned the sale of snake venom for treating MS (or any other disease such as arthritis) until its safety and effectiveness has been scientifically tested. The National Multiple Sclerosis Society has funded laboratory research on honey bee venom, but there is not yet any proof that it is effective.

How Expensive Is It? Both therapies are only moderately expensive. But they are time consuming. Snake venom therapy requires 20 injections. Honey bee therapy requires three sessions a week for six months—with live bees!

Any Dangers? Yes and yes. In both therapies, short-term side effects include pain, inflammation, and swelling at the sting or injection site. Bee stings are obviously painful, but, fortunately, there is now a venom solution that can be injected. Severe allergic reactions have been reported, however, for both therapies. Bee stings can create anaphylactic shock in allergic people; one woman died from a rare type of brain hemorrhage while undergoing snake venom therapy.

YOU'LL KNOW AN ALTERNATIVE THERAPY IS A SCAM IF . . .

- *The physician or advertisement calls it a CURE for MS. Look out for the word "miracle."*
- *The physician or company wants your money up front.*
- *The alternative healthcare provider refuses to work with your regular doctor.*
- *The treatment is based on a "secret formula."*
- *You found out about the therapy via an infomercial, an ad in the back of a magazine, an ad meant to look like the editorial pages of a magazine or newspaper, or solely on the Internet.*
- *Promotional material consists of testimonials from satisfied customers—especially if they only use their initials or first names.*

"An Irritating Itch" or Candida Treatment

What Is It? There is a theory out there stating that yeast infections may trigger exacerbations of multiple sclerosis. The overgrowth of Candida, or yeast fungus, is associated with infections in the mouth (thrush) or the vagina (monilia); people who are susceptible to yeast infections are those who have autoimmune system diseases such as AIDS or who are taking chemotherapy medications or steroids. Since MS also involves the immune system, the theory's supporters believe that people who have the disease are "Candidiasis hypersensitive." The theory also states that this hypersensitivity causes many of the symptoms of MS: fatigue, anxiety, depression, even muscle aches and pains.

To create a more balanced system, healthcare professionals may advise patients to stay away from moldy environments and any foods containing yeast. They might also prescribe vitamin supplements and antifungal drugs such as nystatin, ketoconazole, or amphotericin.

How Effective Is It? Unfortunately, no one knows. There is no evidence to support the fact that the presence of excess candida causes or worsens multiple sclerosis. Nor have clinical studies shown that antifungal agents or diet therapy work.

How Expensive Is It? Costs include doctor visits and the purchase of antifungal drugs and vitamins. Prescription antifungal drugs can be very expensive.

Any Dangers? The risk of this form of therapy is relatively low. A minority of people, however, cannot tolerate antifungal medications; they end up with liver inflammation and, in rare cases, fatal liver damage.

"A Vitamin a Day Keeps the Doctor Away" *or Vitamins, Minerals, Herbs* *and Other Non-Food Supplements*

What Is It? Vitamins, minerals, and herbs are potent stuff. They are a billion-dollar-a-year industry, as mainstream as toothpaste and shampoo. Taking a vitamin a day, or even a series of supplements, might be beneficial to your bones, your heart, your brain, your rate of aging—your general good health. Traditional physicians even recommend certain supplements to their patients.

The tricky part comes from taking supplements in higher quantities. It comes from taking these supplements without supervision. It comes from having a chronic illness that you want to help—especially one that involves your immune system. Why are people with MS drawn to them? Because they are accessible and relatively inexpensive—and they provide the possibility of hope.

Taking these supplements does pose a risk, however, for people who have MS. Many of them stimulate the immune system—which is exactly what you don't want to do. If you have MS, your immune system is already working overtime and has "turned against itself." You want to stick with supplements that may promote nerve health, bone strength, and energy—and stay away from those that pinpoint the immune system.

That general warning aside, there are still so many different kinds of supplements that we cannot examine every single one within the confines of this book. But, to take some of the confusion away, we've listed the more popular supplements, incorporating risks and benefits together under each one. (*Please note that the expense of this complementary therapy varies from supplement to supplement. Check with your local pharmacy or health food store for exact prices.*)

- **The Antioxidant Group: Vitamins A, C, and E and the supplements Pycnogenol and Grape Seed Extract:** There is good news and bad news about these vitamins and supplements. On one hand, they attack free radicals, the free-floating pieces of chemicals that may damage nerve and brain cells. These free radicals may be released by the once-friendly immune cells and attack the myelin that coats your nerve cells; they may also cause axonal injury. But, conversely, these antioxidants help strengthen your immune system—a real plus for people who do not have MS and a real negative for those who do. The best bet? Get these essential vitamins in your multivitamin or take them separately in low doses. This way you get the benefits without the potential downside.

- **Polyunsaturated Fatty Acids: Evening Primrose Oil, Borage Oil, GLA (linoleic acid), and Flaxseed Oil:** People with MS have been found to have a deficiency in polyunsaturated fatty acids (Omega-6 and Omega-3 fatty acids) in their bodies; these fatty acids are a main component of myelin. Further, it is believed by some that these fatty acids slow down the immune system's activity—a real benefit for people with MS. The only negative: These supplements decrease the absorption of Vitamin E— which your body needs in moderate amounts.
- **Blood Balancer: Vitamin B12 (cobalamin):** A common belief among proponents of alternative medicines is that MS is caused, in part, by a deficiency of vitamin B12. Because this vitamin is essential for normal nerve function and red blood cell production, you definitely need to get some every day; a low level may injure your spinal cord and the optic nerves. Normal intake of the eggs, meat, poultry, shellfish, and dairy products usually provides sufficient amounts. If your doctor finds that you have low levels of Vitamin B12 in your bloodstream, she may recommend supplements taken orally or as an injection once a month.

- **Urinary Tract Infection Fighter: Cranberry Juice Capsules:** People who have MS are susceptible to urinary tract infections (UTIs) and anything that can help prevent them is good. Research has shown that cranberry juice makes the lining of the urinary tract too "slippery" for bacteria to cling to its walls. It may also kill the bacteria outright as well. There are no known side effects to taking a cranberry juice capsule, but remember: This is a preventive measure only. If you currently have a UTI, you'll need to see your doctor and take antibiotics.

- **Strong Bones Builder: Calcium:** According to an old theory, calcium was linked to MS. Various studies suggested that MS occurred more in people who drank a lot of milk as children and who dropped their intake suddenly when they became teenagers. But there is no hard evidence to prove these studies correct. Calcium, however, is a good supplement to take to avoid osteoporosis—a condition more common in MS.

- **Depression Fighter: St. John's Wort**: This yellow flower has gained immense popularity as a natural remedy for depression. And studies show that St. John's Wort does work on mildly depressed people. Many people who have MS, however, have more than mild depression and may need a stronger antidepressant. Further, St. John's Wort can weaken your ability to metabolize other drugs, such as amitryptyline (Elavil®), nortriptyline (Pamelor®), Carbamazepine (Tegretol®), phenobarbital, phenytoin (Dilantin®), and primidone (Mysoline®). If you feel depressed enough to consider St. John's Wort, your best bet is to first check with your doctor.

- **Mind Sharpener: Ginkgo Biloba:** This might sound like an exotic fish, but it is, in reality, an antioxidant that has been used to improve cognitive function in China for thousands of years. Studies have also discovered that ginkgo biloba inhibits platelet activating factor (PAF)—which, in turn, decreases the activity of your immune system. However, studies done to test its effectiveness on MS have been contradictory. One study suggested that decreasing immune system function made an MS attack less severe. But another study did not find any difference between people who took ginkgo biloba and those who did not. Even more importantly: Ginkgo biloba has been found to inhibit blood clotting—and cause bleeding disorders. *We strongly recommend staying away from this particular herb, even if you don't have a bleeding disorder.*
- **Energy Builder: Ginseng:** You can find this herb in everything from your ice tea drink to your ice cream. Ginseng, also known as Panax ginseng, has been used in China for thousands of years to enhance physical performance and increase stamina. A natural substance that would fight the fatigue and malaise so common in MS would be wonderful; unfortunately, there is conflicting information about ginseng's efficacy. Not only do some studies show it has no effect on the fatigue caused by MS, but it might actually stimulate the immune system as well something that must be avoided if you have this disease.

"Take a Nice, Deep Breath"
or Hyperbaric Oxygen Treatment (HBO)

What Is It? Utilizing the same type of chamber used when divers have the "bends," this therapy involves breathing oxygen under increased pressure.

How Effective Is It? This "forced oxygen" treatment has been found to work for air embolisms (which divers can get when they swim to the surface too quickly), burn victims, and people with serious wounds. Since it also suppresses immune system activity, HBO was also thought to be a good alternative treatment for MS. Although anecdotal evidence suggests that it may improve MS symptoms in a few patients, scientific studies show that it in no way alters the course of the disease. We cannot recommend HBO as a therapy for MS.

How Expensive Is It? HBO is expensive—timewise and financially. Treatments must be done by a specialist over a period of many weeks—and this doesn't come cheaply. Since there is no scientific proof of HBO's effectiveness, insurance will not cover it as a treatment for MS patients.

Any Dangers? There are no serious problems if it is done at a reputable center, but once again, we cannot recommend this therapy even if you can afford to pay for it yourself.

"Drawn to You" or Magnetotherapy

What Is It? Magnets have been in vogue for helping almost every ailment from arthritis to fatigue. A magnetic field is supposed to improve cell function, circulation, and metabolism. It is also supposed to calm the nervous system and

DIETS TO SUIT EVERY THEORY

Some people believe that various foods may trigger an MS attack. These include milk and dairy products, caffeine, gluten (found in wheat, rye, barley and other grains), ketchup, vinegar, wine, and corn. Is this true? The only way to test it is to eliminate one of these food items from your diet for a prolonged period of time and see if there are any positive effects. (But even then, a beneficial effect can simply be the particular course of your disease—and have nothing to do with diet.) Remember: relapses can last years.

There is also a belief that too many saturated fats can trigger attacks. In theory, a person with MS should eat a diet that's rich in polyunsaturated fats (and Omega 3 and 6 fatty acids) and low in saturated fat. In fact, that's a good diet plan for most people to stay healthy! Some of the diets out there specifically designed for people with MS (named after their "inventor") include:

- The Evers Diet *in which you eat only raw foods.*
- The MacDougal Diet *which is both gluten-free and sugar-free and includes the intake of megavitamins.*
- The Cambridge Diet, *a liquid diet used primarily for the obese.*
- The Swank Diet, *rich in polyunsaturated fats such as safflower, sunflower, olive, and sesame oils; leafy green vegetables; beans; and fish. It also includes vitamin therapy and cod-liver oil supplements. During the first year, people who follow this diet are expected to stay away from red meat.*

In general, a diet supporting overall good health is recommended.

restore balance to your body. Magnetotherapy can involve a wide variety of applications ranging from a magnetic bracelet to a magnetic overlay for your mattress.

How Effective Is It? Do magnets help patients with MS? Probably not. In an Hungarian study of people with chronic but stabilized diseases who received magnetotherapy showed mild to moderate improvement in their spasticity; they also experienced some cognitive and bladder function improvement. Once the treatment stopped, however, so did the improvements (within 4 to 16 weeks). Unfortunately, there are no double-blind scientific studies that have specifically researched people with multiple sclerosis.

How Expensive Is It? Only the cost of the magnets, which are relatively inexpensive and can be found in health stores, mail-order catalogues and magazines, or on the Internet. There is no scientific evidence that favors one type of magnet over another.

Any Dangers? There are no known risks at this time.

"Keep Needling Me" or Acupuncture
What Is It? To accept acupuncture, you must look past the truths about body function we've learned to accept in Western civilization. Used in China and the Far East for centuries, acupuncture deals with the flow of energy (qi) through 14 main pathways (meridians) throughout your body. This energy must flow freely in order to avoid disease. To rebalance your body, trained acupuncturists insert thin, sterilized metal needles into various points on your body. The placement of these needles depends on the problems you are experiencing; different meridians control different bodily functions and balance. If you are phobic to needles, or if the insertion hurts too much, acupressure can be used instead.

Here, a trained professional applies pressure at various points on your body with his thumbs.

How Effective Is It? Nobody quite knows why acupuncture works for various conditions—we just know it does. One theory explains its effectiveness on opiods, chemicals released with the needle's insertion. It is believed that these opiods reduce pain.

Acupuncture has attracted so much attention that the National Institutes of Health set up a 12-member panel in 1997 to evaluate various studies that had been conducted on the subject. It has been found to help people having chemotherapy, surgery, and dental work. But even with this positive reinforcement, there are few studies of the effectiveness of acupuncture on people with MS. A British Columbia survey of people with MS found that about two-thirds of those surveyed experienced a reduction in pain, spasticity, bowel and bladder problems, weakness, balance, tingling, and sleep disorders. Other studies are examining acupuncture's ability to help the depression, anxiety, and dizziness associated with MS. It's important to remember, however, that these studies are inconclusive. More long-term evaluations must be conducted before we can say unequivocally that acupuncture is effective in treating MS.

How Expensive Is It? Acupuncture is usually done once or twice a week in a doctor's office; the cost of each treatment ranges from $45 to $60. It usually takes several weeks for any improvements to be noted.

Any Dangers? The main side effect found in people with MS is a sensitivity to the needles; they have experienced pain at the site of insertion. Many of them have also experienced drowsiness after a session.

There are many more alternative medicines that have been used to stave off MS symptoms and halt its reoccurrence. To find out more, we suggest you contact any of the addresses you'll find in the back of this book.

But one final cautionary note: There are highly effective medicines available today that are scientifically *proven* to modify the course of MS. Never abandon one of these proven therapies in favor of CAM alone. If you desire, use CAM exactly as it is intended—as a complementary approach to proven therapies. Remember: the more you know, the more empowered you will be. You will be able to find real hope—not exploitation.

Our journey is almost at an end. But there is still one more arena that we have not yet talked about: your family and society at large. Let's visit them now.

CHAPTER SIXTEEN

MS AND YOUR FAMILY, YOUR JOB, AND THE WORLD AT LARGE

At first, I was afraid to tell the people at work that I had MS. I was afraid they'd start treating me differently, as if I was sick. I was afraid I'd be passed over for promotion. Well, guess what? That didn't happen. People showed love and concern—and my boss even made it clear to tell him if and when I'd need to have my office modified. What a relief!

—A 38-year-old male lawyer
with relapsing-remitting MS

Claire was 18 when she got married. Charlie was her first love, the guy she dated in high school and has been with ever since. Claire was supposed to go to college after graduation, but she got pregnant. Charlie and she married and within three years had two kids. Although they didn't choose the lives they had, they did okay. There was no real passionate love, no feelings that they were soulmates, but they survived—as so many people do. Claire took care of the house and the kids, both teenagers now, and Charlie took care of the finances. He had a thriving accounting firm, and he worked hard to keep it that way.

The children, one girl and one boy, came to rely on their mother for emotional support; Charlie was either too busy working or too distant. It's not that he didn't care, he just didn't know how. He was cold, distant, more comfortable with numbers than feelings.

Things would have gone on the way they had for 16 years if Claire hadn't gotten sick. When she was 34 years old, she suddenly developed slurred speech and a loss of coordination. A few days later, she also noticed numbness in her legs.

It was time to visit her doctor.

After a thorough examination, the doctor decided to refer her to a neurologist. He had an MRI performed and sure enough, the MRI showed multiple lesions. The diagnosis? Multiple sclerosis.

The course of her disease was worrisome: She might have a progressive form of multiple sclerosis with symptoms that may become debilitating. No one knew how the disease would "play out", no one knew if she'd improve—or by how much—after this particular episode.

Suddenly, just like that, the pillar of strength in the family, the emotional anchor, had disappeared. In her place was this worried, anxious stranger—who was terrified she'd become dependent on her family.

Unfortunately, Claire's worst fears became true several months later. Her symptoms—her speech and balance problems and her numbness—returned at full throttle; she couldn't walk and her ability to communicate decreased even more.

This time around, Claire had to spend several weeks in a rehabilitation hospital where she'd had physical therapy to strengthen her legs and exercises to improve her speech. The therapies helped a great deal, but not enough for Claire to return to her old routines. She was told she would need continued rehabilitation on an outpatient basis. She would also need a caregiver at home.

Alas, home was no longer the safe, secure, mundane place it was only a few months ago. In addition to a caregiver who came to the house five days a week, the children had to pitch in and help. They hated having to take care of their mother; they hated the role reversal. They resented having to miss parties and football games, or just hanging out with their friends. It made them feel awful to have to cook dinner and do chores around the house; it made them angry that their mom wasn't available, that she couldn't be a part of the carpool and pick them up at the mall. Guilt, anger, sadness, and pain: A potent combination of emotions was brewing just under the surface.

Charlie's emotional state was worse. He'd always had poor coping skills and had relied on his wife to take care of things. He just couldn't handle the anxiety and fear he felt; the responsibility felt like lead. Instead of helping his kids, he pushed them away. In fact, he pushed everything away. He escaped to his office more and more. Whatever intimacy Charlie and Claire had shared was gone. In its place were two resentful strangers sharing a bed.

This family needed help—and fast.

It came first from the school counselor. Concerned about the teenagers' sudden drop in grades and their out-of-character aggressiveness, she had Charlie and Claire come into school.

The family needed therapy, both together and alone. Claire had already been seeing a counselor as an outpatient at the rehabilitation hospital, but no one else in the family wanted to "open up" to a stranger.

Charlie was the worst. He'd never voiced his feelings to anyone. He didn't want to start now, especially to someone who might know "all about him" from his wife!

After some convincing, Charlie agreed to see a family therapist, someone who was a stranger to everyone. After all,

Charlie had to face the fact that his family was in trouble, that the dynamics had changed, that staying late at the office wouldn't solve anything. They all needed to recognize their anger and confusion—and learn how to cope with their brave new world.

Three years later, the family is intact. They will never be that perfect nuclear family depicted in television ads, but they have learned to live with MS, and they have learned how to cope with their feelings—and the disease itself. Thanks to the disease-modifying drug Claire took, the progression slowed down; she was able to be more independent with certain adaptations. The two teens are in college—one a sophomore, the other a freshman—and they are enjoying their new life.

And Charlie? He's learned to open up and talk to his wife. Ironically, the MS brought the family together. It brought intimacy back to their marriage. Happily ever after? Maybe not. But happily for now would do just fine.

This story illuminates just how serious multiple sclerosis is—on the family. The impact of the disease is felt not just by the patient, but by the spouse or partner, the children, the friends, even the colleagues at work. Multiple sclerosis is a family disease. It involves everyone within the patient's circle.

And, like Claire and Charlie, people need to learn how to accept change, cope with new feelings, and change the shape of the circle to fit a whole new way of doing things.

This chapter provides some insights and suggestions for families, friends, and co-workers. It also provides disability awareness for people and places outside the patient's close circle.

IT REALLY IS ALL IN THE FAMILY

The first harsh truth: When your loved one has been diagnosed with MS, your life will change. Even if the disease takes a mild course and relapses are few and far between, MS will affect you in some way for the rest of your life. When will it strike again? Will it be worse this time? As I've reiterated time and again throughout this book, you have to learn to live with uncertainty. And, as always, the best way to do this is "to hope for the best, but prepare for the worst."

This doesn't have to be "death sentence," a grim destiny for everyone involved. No, it just means taking care of the very practical financial concerns—and the more ambiguous emotional scenarios. It means being prepared.

The two key words are support and information. Together, they can help everyone cope better.

Helpline #1: Organizing Your Finances

First, the good news: Most people who are diagnosed with MS do not develop such severe disabilities that they need care 24/7. But because there is no real way to predict the course of MS, it's best to have everything in order—and to have everyone know what that "order" is. In fact, this is common sense advice for anyone—MS or not. Whether it's investment portfolios, income tax returns, retirement savings plans, money market funds, life and disability insurance, or both living and after-death wills, talk to your accountant or financial advisor to ensure that both you and your family know exactly what is going on.

Helpline #2: Insurance Issues

Medical insurance becomes crucial when you are diagnosed with MS. Find out exactly what your insurance covers—including primary and secondary insurance policies and whether you are eligible for Medicare. Find out what Social Security benefits your family can expect when you can no longer work. Check to see if you have private disability insurance; many people don't realize that they are covered by their employer. Talk to the rehabilitation hospital's case manager about these important issues. She can help you make informed decisions—as well as determine what your options are.

Helpline #3: Budgeting for the Future

No one has a crystal ball, but we all at least try to save for our eventual retirement. If you have been diagnosed with MS, it's even more important to save for the future. Sit down with a paper and pencil and discuss your finances with your spouse. Determine what you need to live on every month—from mortgage payments to dry cleaning bills—and see how you can cut back if necessary. Try to put more into your savings account. Think of it this way: Even if your disease remains mild, the money won't go to waste in your "golden years!"

Helpline #4: Know Your Rights

Make sure that you and your spouse are familiar with the Americans with Disabilities Act (ADA) that became law in 1990—as well as other acts of Congress that can help provide for housing, transportation, and employment for people with disabilities. You might be entitled to a certain amount of money each week. You might be provided with outside help—easing the strain on your family. Ask. Learn. You won't know anything until you do.

Helpline #5: Know Thyself—and Everyone Else in the Family

There's an old expression: "The road to hell is paved with good intentions." Your family might be very willing to take charge: Make dinner, tend to your transferring needs, help you dress, and drive you where you need to go. The reality, however, may be very different from the loving fantasy.

Think about it. Perhaps you are the husband and your wife has always taken care of all the household chores and errands. Like Claire in our earlier example, she did everything that involved the home. Then, suddenly, the diagnosis comes in. Perhaps she begins to deteriorate, perhaps she needs a wheelchair, perhaps she needs to slow down her pace. It doesn't matter what her condition is. What does matter is that something has changed. Your life has changed. Emotions may play havoc as you begin to help around the house. There's the guilt you may feel because you can walk around, do ten things at once, have a burst of energy—while the woman you love has to take a nap. Then there's the anger that builds up. Suddenly, you don't see the friends you used to visit; you don't go out to dinner; you don't laugh. In fact, it seems like the only thing you talk about is your wife's disease and how she is feeling. This resentment can grow even greater as the pressures from your job mount, as stress and exhaustion take their toll. And, to add insult to injury, there's your wife getting all the attention from your relatives, from the friends who stop by, even from the local pharmacist!

Role reversal, which started out with such high hopes, has become a vicious cycle of anger, resentment, and guilt—which has broken up more than one marriage.

How to cope? Simple: seek help and information. Talk to your case manager at the rehabilitation hospital. Talk to the your wife's counselor. Begin your own individual therapy.

On another level, figure out what you can spend on an outside caregiver—and have that caregiver do many of the chores. And, if you can't afford outside service, it still doesn't mean that you have to be miserable. Count on your friends and families. See who can help you and when. Don't be afraid to ask for help. Most people want to help. Most people like the feeling of being needed. Reach out.

GOOD WILL HOSTING

The last thing you might feel like doing is playing host to your friends or family when your wife or husband is experiencing an MS flare-up. You feel depressed, scared, and completely stressed out. But, believe it or not, a party might be just what you need. Studies have found that caregivers who get lots of visitors have less stress than those who never hear the doorbell ring.

Entertaining doesn't mean competing with Martha Stewart—or even the Joneses who live next door. You can make simple sandwiches or serve ice tea, soda, and chips and dip. Better yet, have your guests bring a dish that everyone can share. An added plus: Your loved one will enjoy the company, too.

Helpline # 6: Mending Fences with the Kids

Role reversal will not just frighten you—it can hurt your children. As they see their mother or father deteriorate, they can become irrationally angry and scared. Even if their parent has remitting-relapsing MS, there is always that uncertainty: "Is Mom going to wake up this morning with that funny walk?" If you notice that grades are beginning to drop, that behavior in school and at home has become more aggressive, that your children spend too much time incommunicado behind their bedroom doors or that they spend too much time away from home, it spells trouble.

Then there's the embarrassment they might feel about their parent's illness—and the guilt that the shame creates. They don't want to bring their friends over after school because mom might be watching television in her wheelchair but, on the other hand, they are angry at themselves for feeling this way.

Children can also go in the opposite direction. Instead of avoiding the issue, they face it head-on—and ignore their growing-up years. Instead of trying out for the school play, they are home making dinner. Instead of going to the soccer game, they are making mom's bed. Instead of going away to college, they are hanging out at home, alert to any help their parent might need. This is just as bad as anger in children; both will affect them adversely. They need to know that there's a balance between helping out—and helping themselves out.

What to do? Again, help and information are key. Talk to the school guidance counselor. Try to talk to your kids. And make sure that they start either family therapy with you or individual one-on-one therapy.

LET'S HEAR IT FOR THE CAREGIVER: TIME OUT!

Stress is insidious. The more stress caregivers feel internally, the more they'll get externally. A chronic disease is a definite source of stress—on the person with MS and on everyone around him. The trouble is that everyone expects the person with MS to feel stressed, to feel anxious and afraid. Not so his spouse or his kids. But just as he needs top-grade care, so does each family member. If you are a caregiver, make sure you take time out for yourself—doing something completely selfish, just for you. Maybe it's going to a movie. Maybe it's settling down with a good book. Or maybe it's taking a solitary walk in the woods. Have one of your friends or relatives help out while you pursue your own interests a few hours a week. You'll come back refreshed, revitalized, and much better able to take care of your loved one who has MS.

Helpline #7: Poor Me

It's understandable that you may feel like a victim. It makes sense that the fact that you have MS can make you depressed, anxious, and even put you in a state of denial. (*See Chapter 12 for more information on depression and MS.*) But these same feelings can also affect your family. It's also easy to feel like a victim when you feel as if you are making a "sacrifice," spending more time tending your sick spouse, parent, or child than you do on the more "normal" routines of everyday life. If you start having feelings of hopelessness and helplessness, STOP! Seek out professional help. It's not easy living with someone who has a chronic disease. Talk to your family doctor or the rehabilitation hospital's counselor. Find out about support groups in your area from your local Y or community center. You can also find information and help for a caregiver's depression and emotional health from the National Multiple Sclerosis Society. (*See the appendix in the back of this book for the address.*)

WORKING OUT

The family circle isn't the only place where help and information are crucial. Disability awareness also goes with you on the job. The workplace, the office where you go every day, can be either a source of pleasure—or more frustration.

Some questions—and answers—for ensuring productivity and respect on the job.

Work-Related Issue #1: Do I have to tell my boss?

Not necessarily. Some people prefer keeping it quiet—until they've had several relapses and the symptoms are obvious to everyone. But when that occurs, your boss can wonder why you didn't say something before; he might be more upset than if you'd come forward and told him. He might feel a sense of betrayal. In other words, waiting can backfire in your face.

There is no right or wrong answer. It all depends on the culture in your particular workplace. But if you do decide to speak up, be clear and upfront. Talk to your boss or your human resources department. Tell them exactly what is going on and what you are doing to keep your disease at bay. Some hints:

1. Arrange for a meeting in advance; don't leave it up to chance. Arrive on time and wear business-like clothes.
2. Write down what you want to say beforehand. Practice at home to ensure you will be confident and direct. Emotion won't help your case.
3. Use language that is straightforward and positive—not defensive or belligerent. Use words like "we . . .", "together, perhaps we can . . .", "it makes sense for both of us . . .". Answer any questions with honesty. Be direct and make eye contact.
4. Stay upbeat. If you act defensive, depressed, or anxious, your boss or human resource representative will have second thoughts. If you bring optimism, as well as solutions to enhance your productivity on the job, your situation will look much better.
5. It's important to keep things in perspective. Most companies want to help; your boss will most likely react with kindness and an offer to help. But, if necessary, remember the Americans with Disabilities Act requires your workplace to accommodate many disabilities. The law may be on your side.

Work-Related Issue #2: How do I make my office compatible with my disability?

This is an easy one. The ADA has already mapped out the ways your workplace can adapt to people with disabilities.

If you are weak and have trouble entering and leaving your office, the company can restructure its facilities; it can provide an electronic door opener for you.

If you've lost strength in your lower extremities, your company can make provisions to ensure you do more work at your desk instead of running around to meetings. Aisles, elevators, and doorways should already be wide enough to provide for wheelchairs: It's the law.

If you're too tired to last a full day, you might be able to have your work schedule modified to fit in breaks; you may also be able to do some work via telecommunication from home.

If your problems with coordination and balance interfere with your job, request a reassignment to a different position. There may be other positions available in your place of business. But always keep in mind: Your employer only has to make reasonable accommodations, and you need to have the skills and abilities to perform the alternate job.

If you have problems with your eyes, with hand-eye coordination, or with some cognitive skills, a specially adapted computer can be installed with a foot pedal that will move your cursor. You can keep your Palm Pilot or any other appointment software program on screen so you'll know what you have to do—and when—each day.

Work-Related Issue #3: How Do I Handle Discrimination?

Let's face it. Get a group of people together and you will always find one or two individuals who will be jealous of anyone who gets ahead or is successful—except themselves, of course. It wouldn't matter if the successful person had three chins, looked like Julia Roberts—or had a disability. There will always be people who complain.

When it comes to a worker with a disability, however, there is a bit more subtlety involved. The resentment among co-workers usually comes in the form of pity: The person with a disability was promoted because her supervisor felt sorry for her.

THE POWER OF YOU

Never underestimate personal empowerment. By taking charge of the things you can control, you will become stronger, more confident, and more positive in your outlook on life. How do you get that empowerment? One way is to try the suggestions offered in this chapter. Another is to think of the ways you can better serve yourself. For example, doctor visits are a part of your life. Although you can't totally control the course of your disease or when you might need to go to the doctor, you can write down your questions in advance. You can have someone go with you to "catch" information you might not hear—and to help ease your anxiety. And, if you get tired in the afternoon, you can book your appointments early in the day.

Other roads to personal empowerment? Start a healthier lifestyle. Join that aqua aerobics class you've been thinking about for the past few months (but make sure it is given in a cool pool). Buy those exotic-looking fruits and vegetables you've been eyeing every time you go to the store. Sample whole-grain products—you just might like them. Check out travel organizations, such as Flying Wheels and Mobility International, specifically designed for people with disabilities; they can make traveling much easier—and enhance your enjoyment. (See the appendix for addresses and phone numbers.) *Doing things that help yourself will indeed help you.*

The only way to keep office gossip at bay is to make sure that if you have a disability, your work is well done and your performance exemplary. It would be difficult to elicit pity when you are upbeat and professional. And if you happen to be the supervisor responsible for the promotion, make sure that you did it, not as a sign of pity, but as worth. Hire, promote, and fire based on merit—and you won't have to fear any second-guessing or "talk."

Work-Related Issue # 4: As an employer, do I see a possible lawsuit in my future?

It's possible, and very probable, that the first woman who applied for a job could have shouted "Sex discrimination!" The same holds true for different ethnic backgrounds and race. Discrimination is an insidious form of prejudice. It prevents people who are highly qualified and able to contribute a great deal to the workplace from getting jobs. That's why discrimination laws were created—and why they protect potential workers from not being hired because of the color of their skin, their gender—or their disabilities.

But discrimination is cloudy today. Excuses can be made; other reasons given for termination. And discrimination can be overused—by both employers and employees. You cannot look inside a crystal ball to see whether that woman (whom you only met twice) will surprise you with a sexual harassment suit—or whether that man (who looks 20 years younger than you) will sue you for age discrimination. The best advice? Go by the books, hire and fire by ability, and give appropriate counseling and fair warning.

Most people are not vindictive—and that includes people with disabilities. If they get a warning at work, they will try hard to change any unsatisfactory behavior. And if let go, they will act as any able-bodied person would.

Human diversity makes tolerance more than a virtue; it makes it a requirement for survival.

— Rene Dubois

PUBLIC SCENES

The home and the office are not the only places where a dose of disability awareness wouldn't hurt. In the same way your family or your co-workers might react to your MS, so, too, might strangers. You know where to go for help in the home. You know your rights and privileges in the workplace. But there's one more arena that needs to be treated with sensitivity: public places.

Being seen out in public is exactly that: being seen. Although most of us are not movie stars who are used to our every move being watched, we are still, at some level, on display when we go out to dinner, spend an evening at the theater, or attend a cocktail party. We shouldn't burp or use dental floss in public. We shouldn't lick our soup bowls or eat with our fingers.

Although the course of your MS might not create disabilities that are immediately noticed in public, it's important for both you and those in your world to develop disability etiquette awareness when you are "outside." Whether a one-on-one introduction or a group gathering, disability etiquette awareness is as important for preserving the respect and dignity of the people around you as the polite behavior your parents taught you when you were young. In short, you need to know how to act in public settings—whether you are the person with the disability or not.

Here is a list of "public concerns" that would do Emily Post proud. They involve common sense—and a dose of sensitivity. Use them yourself—and pass them along to the people in your life. They can make all the difference between feeling good about yourself—or self-conscious and sad. And the best part? These "rules of etiquette" are easy and simple to implement. They take less time than, well, flossing your teeth!

Disability Awareness and the Public at Large

- *Don't order food for someone with a disability:* He is completely capable of ordering his own.
- *Avoid being over-solicitous:* This means talking too loudly, micro-managing her every move, and, yes, cutting her food in a restaurant! These behaviors, even though they stem from kindness, will backfire—making a person with a disability embarrassed and feeling about six years old to boot!
- *Plan ahead.* If you are going out on the town, call the concert hall or theater ahead of time. If you are going with someone with a hearing disability, see if closed-caption, hearing amplification, or binoculars are available. Find out how and where the accessible facilities are located. This way everyone in your party will be able to get to your seats as smoothly as everyone else.

> *I celebrate myself and sing myself.*
>
> — Walt Whitman

- *Don't use your disability—or your friend's disability—to get special treatment:* A disability doesn't give you "celebrity status." You shouldn't get the best seats—or a chance to go backstage. The goal of disability awareness is ordinary equality. In other words, people with disabilities are no better or worse than anyone else.
- *Don't leave a person with a disability alone at the table when everyone else is on the floor dancing:* No one likes being a wallflower, whether able-bodied or a person with a disability. And, besides, almost everyone likes to dance!
- *Offer to get a drink or a plate of appetizers for a person with a disability—but only if you are going to the buffet table yourself.* It's always nice to be considerate, but you don't want to be overbearing.
- *Don't raise your voice.* It doesn't help when you meet someone from a foreign country—and it isn't necessary when you meet someone with a disability.
- *Extend your hand as you would meeting anyone during an introduction.* Even people with prosthetic devices will find it polite.
- *Avoid acts of pity.* Compassion is one thing but "high drama" is another. If you happen to be able-bodied, don't tell the person with a disability that you just couldn't cope with the situation if it had happened to you.

TAKE ME FOR A DRIVE

Driving is considered a "God-given right." From the first day we get our permits at 16, we recognize our ability to drive as a sign of freedom. Unfortunately, your MS could very well affect your ability to drive. Recognize that it is your condition—not your value as a human being—that is creating problems. Don't wait until you have an accident or, God forbid, hit someone and kill her. If you sense that your driving is not what it used to be—either because of mobility issues, double vision, or cognitive problems—talk to your physician. She can have your driving skills re-evaluated, and you can find out if you are safe to drive. Like not drinking and driving, ensuring your safety and that of those you love is the responsible way of handling things.

These specific suggestions are only that: suggestions. If you think about it, there are probably countless more daily courtesies you can perform with a friend, a co-worker, or family member who is disabled. And, if you are disabled, there are countless courtesies that the people in your life can show you as well. Remember: A great deal of awareness is common sense. Add a dash of informed behavior and a dose of kindness and you have it all. Or as it was said many centuries ago: "*Do unto others as you would have done unto you.*"

LIVING SUCCESSFULLY
WITH MULTIPLE SCLEROSIS

How did you react when you heard you had MS? Most likely, you were angry and sad and depressed all at once. You were confused and shocked.

This is understandable—and entirely appropriate. Anyone in the same circumstances would act the same way. The good news is that you will bounce back. Research shows that although your self-esteem may be seriously affected by your disease, you will most likely regain your sense of self-worth—even when you experience a relapse.

Research also shows that people with multiple sclerosis want information—the more the better. And the more information they gather, the more resilient and in control they become.

We hope that this book has helped you in that quest. We hope it has answered some questions and led the way to others which you will want to discuss with your doctor, your counselor, your support group, or simply explore on your own on the Internet.

Is there a cure for MS? No. Is there a way to slow down its progression? Absolutely. Every year new medications and new therapies are introduced. In 2001 alone, the National Multiple Sclerosis Society committed $30 million to new research projects to help reduce the impact of multiple sclerosis.

Information, help—and new hope—are within reach.

Life isn't always fair. No one gets away scot-free. But accepting your condition is the first step toward a better tomorrow, a better outlook, a better quality of life.

You can live with multiple sclerosis. Even more importantly, you can live well.

NAMES, ADDRESSES, AND WEBSITES OF HELPFUL ORGANIZATIONS

Alliance for Technology Access
2175 E. Francisco Blvd., Suite L
San Raphael, CA 94901
(415) 455-4575
www.atacess.org

American Association of People with Disabilities
1819 H Street, NW, Suite 330
Washington, DC 20006
(800) 840-8844
(202) 457-8168
(202) 457-0473 (fax)
www.aapd.com

American Occupational Therapy Association
4720 Montgomery Lane
P. O. Box 31220
Bethesda, MD 20824-1220
(301) 652-2682
www.aota.org

Association for Persons with Severe Handicaps
29 West Susquehanna Avenue, Suite 210
Baltimore, MD 21204
(410) 828-8274
(410) 828-6706 (fax)
www.tash.org

American Physical Therapy Association
1111 North Fairfax Street
Alexandria, VA 22314
(800) 999-2782
www.apta.org

American Speech-Language-Hearing Association
10801 Rockville Pike
Rockville, MD 20852
(800) 498-2071
www.asha.org

Association of Rehabilitation Nurses
4700 West Lake Avenue
Glenview, IL 60025-1485
(800) 229-7530
www.rehabnurse.org

Berlex Laboratories, Inc.
340 Changebridge Road
P. O. Box 1000
Montville, NJ 07045-1000
(973) 487-2000
or:
6 West Belt Road
Wayne, NJ 07420-6806
(973) 694-4100
or:
2600 Hilltop Drive
Richmond, CA 94806
(510) 262-5000
(888) BERLEX4
(800) 788-1467 (*helpline*)
www.berlex.com
www.betaseron.com
Makers of Betaseron

Biogen, Inc.
14 Cambridge Center
Cambridge, MA 02142
(617) 679-2000
(617) 679-2617
www.biogen.com
www.avonex.com
www.msactivesource.com
www.understandingms.com
Makers of Avonex

Center for Applied Special Technology (CAST)
39 Cross Street
Peabody, MA 01960
(508) 531-8555
(508) 531-0192
www.cast.org

DateAble International
35 Wisconsin Circle, Suite 205
Chevy Chase, MD 20815
(301) 656-8723
www.dateable.org
A dating service by and for the disabled

Disability Rights Education and Defense Fund, Inc.
Main Office:
2212 Sixth Street
Berkeley, CA 94710
(510) 644-2555
(510) 841-8645 (fax)
Government Affairs:
1629 K Street, NW, Suite 802
Washington, DC 20006
(202) 986-0375
(202) 775-7465 (fax)
www.dredf.org

Flying Wheels Travel
(A division of Travel Headquarters, Inc.)
143 W. Bridge Street
Owatonna, MN 55060
(507) 451-5005
(507) 451-1684 (fax)
www.flyingwheelstravel.com
E-mail: thq@ll.net
Travel agency for the disabled community

HealthSouth
One HealthSouth Parkway
Birmingham, AL 35243
(800) 765-4772
www.HealthSouth.com

HealthSouth Rehabilitation Institute of San Antonio (RIOSA)
9119 Cinnamon Hill
San Antonio, TX 78240
(210) 691-0737
www.HealthSouth.com

Information Center for Individuals with Disabilities
29 Stanhope Street
Boston, MA 02116
(617) 450-9888
www.disability.net

Job Accommodation Network
P. O. Box 6080
Morgantown, WV 26506-5407
(800) 526-7234 (United States)
(304) 293-7186 (Worldwide)
(304) 293-5407
www.janweb.iedi.wvu.edu
Job information for the disabled

Joint Commission on Accreditation of Healthcare Organizations
(JCAHO)
One Renaissance Boulevard
Oakbrook Terrace, IL 60181
(630) 792-5000
(630) 792-5001
www.jcaho.org

Microsoft Accessibility
www.microsoft.com/enable/
Computer accessibility information for the disabled

Mobility International USA
P. O. Box 10767
Eugene, OR 97440
(541) 343-1284
(541) 343-6812 (fax)
www.miusa.org
Travel accommodations and information

National Center for Disability Services
201 I. U. Willets Road
Albertson, NY 11507-1599
(516) 747-5400
(516) 746-3298 (fax)
www.ncds.org

North Coast Medical
18305 Sutter Boulevard
Morgan Hill, CA 95037-2845
(800) 821-9319
www.ncmedical.com
A good source for medical devices and assistive equipment

National Council of the Disabled
1331 F Street, NW, Suite 1050
Washington, DC 20004
(202) 272-2004
(202) 272-2022 (fax)
www.ned.gov

National Council on Independent Living (NCIL)
1916 Wilson Blvd., Suite 209
Arlington, VA 22201
(703) 525-3406
(703) 525-3400 (fax)
www.ncil.org
A grassroots advocacy group for the disabled

National Library Services for the Blind and Physically
   Handicapped
1291 Taylor Street, NW
Washington, DC 20542
(202) 707-5100
www.loc.gov/nls

National Multiple Sclerosis Society
733 Third Avenue
New York, NY 10017
(212) 986-3240
(212)986-7981
(800) FIGHT MS (344-4867)
www.nmss.org
E-mail: info@nmss.org
Find your local chapter, address, and phone number on website

National Rehabilitation Information Center
1010 Wayne Avenue, Suite 800
Silver Spring, MD 20910
(800) 346-2742
www.naric.com/naric

Paralyzed Veterans of America
801 18th Street, N.W.
Washington, DC 20006-3517
(800) 424-8200
www.pva.org

Rolyan/AbilityOne Corporation
4 Sammons Court
Boilingbrook, IL 60440-4289
(800) 558-8633
(630) 226-5050
(630) 226-1390 (fax)
www.rolyan.com
A good source for medical devices and assistive equipment

Serono, Inc.
100 Longwater Circle
Norwell, MA 02061
(781) 982-9000
(781) 871-6754 (fax)
www.serono.com
www.rebif.com
www.mslifelines.com
www.mstalklive.com
Makers of Rebif

Superintendent of Documents
P. O. Box 371954
Pittsburgh, PA 15250-7054
(866) 512-1800
(202) 512-1800
(202) 512-2250 (fax)
E-mail: gpoaccess@gpo.gov
www.bookstore.gpo.gov
*Documents available on disability law, health insurance, and
the physically challenged*

Teva Neuroscience, Inc.
901 E. 104th Street, Suite 900
Kansas City, MO 64131
(800) 221-4026
(816) 508-5000
(816) 508-5016 (fax)
(800) 887-8100 (helpline)
www.tevamarion.com
www.tevaneuroscience.com
www.copaxone.com
www.mswatch.com
Makers of Copaxone

World Institute on Disability
510 16th Street, Suite 100
Oakland, CA 94612-1500
(510) 763-4100
(510) 763-4109 (fax)
www.wid.org

BIBLIOGRAPHY

Bain, Lisa J., with Randall T. Schapiro, M.D., *Managing MS Through Rehabilitation*, New York: National Multiple Sclerosis Society 2001.

Bever, C.T., Jr., "Multiple Sclerosis: Symptomatic Treatment," *Current Treatment Options in Neurology*, July 1999, Vol. 1, No. 3.

Barnes, David, *Multiple Sclerosis: Questions and Answers*, Coral Springs, FL: Merit Publishing International 2000.

Bowling, Allen C., M.D., Ph.D., *Alternative Medicine and Multiple Sclerosis*, New York: Demos Medical Publishing 2001.

Bowling, Allen, C., M.D., Ph.D., and Thomas Stewart, J.D., PA-C, *Vitamins, Minerals, and Herbs in MS: An Introduction*, New York: National Multiple Sclerosis Society 2000.

Brown, Sharon M., *So You Have Progressive MS?* New York: National Multiple Sclerosis Society 2000.

Carroll, David L., and Jon Dudley Dorman, M.D., *Living Well with MS: A Guide for Patient, Caregiver, and Family*, New York: HarperPerennial 1993.

Clanet, M.G., and D. Brassat, "The Management of Multiple Sclerosis Patients," *Current Opinions in Neurology*, June 2000, Vol. 13, No. 3.

Cooper, Laura D., Esq., and Nancy Law, L.S.W., with Jane Sarnoff, *ADA and People with MS: A Guarantee of Full Participation in Society*, New York: National Multiple Sclerosis Society 1998.

Cavallo, Pamela, with Martha Jablow, *When a Parent has MS: A Teenager's Guide*, New York: National Multiple Sclerosis Society 1997.

Dougherty, Karla and Richard C. Senelick, M.D., *A Baby Boomer's Guide to Women's Health*, Birmingham, AL: HealthSouth Press 2003.

Eastwood, Abe, Ph.D., "Genes and Ms Susceptibility," *Inside MS*, 1999, Vol. 10, No. 1

Frankel, Debra, M.S., O.T.R., with Hettie Jones, *Living with MS*, New York: National Multiple Sclerosis Society 1998.

Foley, Frederick, Ph.D., with Jane Sarnoff, *Taming Stress in Multiple Sclerosis*, New York: National Multiple Sclerosis Society 1998.

Foster, Virginia, *Choosing a Pharmacy Service*, New York: National Multiple Sclerosis Society 1996.

Foster, Virginia, with contribution by Ellen Burstein MacFarlane, *Clear Thinking About Alternative Therapies*, New York: National Multiple Sclerosis Society 2000.

Freeman, J.A., Ph.D., W. Langdon, Ph.D., J.C. Hobart, MRCP, and A.J. Thompson, FRCP, "Inpatient Rehabilitation in Multiple Sclerosis," *Neurology*, 1999, Vol. 52, No. 50.

Freeman, J.A., Ph.D., W. Langdon, Ph.D., J.C. Hobart, MRCP, and A.J. Thompson, FRCP, "The Impact of Inpatient Rehabilitation on Progressive Multiple Sclerosis," *Annals of Neurology*, August 1997, Vol. 42, No. 2.

Gibson, Beth E., P.T., *Stretching for People with MS: An Illustrated Manual*, New York: National Multiple Sclerosis Society 2000.

Popper, Jackie Girsky and Gina Minielli Gunkel, *Incidental Heroes: Disabling the Myths About Multiple Sclerosis*, New York: National Multiple Sclerosis Society 1999.

Hample, Henry, "Depression: The Doctors Are In," *InsideMS*, Spring 2000, Vol.18, No. 2.

Harmon, Jane E., OTR, *At Home with MS: Adapting Your Environment*, New York: National Multiple Sclerosis Society 1997.

Harmon, Mary, *Exercise as Part of Everyday Life*, New York: National Multiple Sclerosis Society 1999.

Holland, Nancy J., R.N., Ed.D., *Controlling Bladder Problems in Multiple Sclerosis*, New York: National Multiple Sclerosis Society 1999.

Holland, Nancy J., R.N., Ed.D., and Robin Frames, *Understanding Bowel Problems in MS*, New York: National Multiple Sclerosis Society 1997.

Holland, Nancy J., R.N., Ed.D., with Serena Stockwell, *Controlling Spasticity*, New York: National Multiple Sclerosis Society 1997.

Jaffee, Cyrisse, Debra Frankel, Barbara LaRoche, and Patricia Dick, *Someone You Know Has Multiple Sclerosis: A Book for Families*, New York: National Multiple Sclerosis Society 1998.

Kalb, Rosalind C., Ph.D., *Multiple Sclerosis: A Guide for Families*, New York: Demos Medical Publishing 1998.

Ko-Ko, C., "Effectiveness of Rehabilitation for Multiple Sclerosis," *Clinical Rehabilitation*, 1999, Vol. 13, Supplement 1.

Kraft, G. H., "Rehabilitation Still the Only Way to Improve Function in Multiple Sclerosis," *Lancet*, December 1999, Vol. 11, No. 354.

Kraft, George H., M.D., and Marci Catanzaro, R.N., Ph.D., *Living with Multiple Sclerosis: A Wellness Approach*, New York: Demos Medical Publishing, Inc. 2000.

La Rocca, Nicholas, G., Ph.D., with Martha King, *Solving Cognitive Problems*, New York: National Multiple Sclerosis Society 1998.

Lander, David L., *Fall Down Laughing*, New York: Jeremy P. Tarcher 2000.

Lockette, Kevin F., and Ann M. Keyes, with The Rehabilitation Institute of Chicago, *Conditioning with Physical Disabilities*, *Champaign*, IL: Human Kinetics 1994.

Langdon, D.W., and A.J. Thompson, "Multiple Sclerosis: A Preliminary Study of Selected Variables Affecting Rehabilitation Outcome," *Multiple Sclerosis*, April 1999, Vol. 5, No. 2.

Minden, Sarah L., M.D., and Debra Frankel, M.S., OTR, *PlainTalk: A Booklet About MS for Families*, New York: National Multiple Sclerosis Society 2001.

O'Connor, Paul, M.D., *Multiple Sclerosis: The Facts You Need*, Buffalo, NY: Firefly Books 1999.

Paralyzed Veterans of America, *Multiple Sclerosis: A Self-Care Guide to Wellness*, ed. by Nancy J. Holland, R.N., Ed.D., and June Halper, M.S.N., R.N., C.S., A.N.P, Washington, DC: Paralyzed Veterans of America June 1998.

Paralyzed Veterans of America, *Fatigue: What You Should Know: A Guide for People with Multiple Sclerosis*, developed by the Multiple Sclerosis Council for Clinical Practice Guidelines, New York: National Multiple Sclerosis Society 2000.

Petajan, J.H., and A.T. White, "Recommendations for Physical Activity in Patients with Multiple Sclerosis," *SportsMedicine*, March 1999, Vol. 27, No. 3.

Polman, Chris H., M.D., Alan J. Thompson, M.D., FRCP, FRCPI, T. Jock Murray, O.C., M.D., FRCPC, MACP, FRCP, and W. Ian McDonald, M.B., Ph.D., FRCP, FmedSci, *Multiple Sclerosis: The Guide to Treatment and Management 5th Edition*, New York: Demos Medical Publishing, Inc. 2001.

Ponichtera-Mulcare, J.A., "Exercise and Multiple Sclerosis," *Medical Science and Sports Exercise*, 1993, Vol. 25, No. 4.

Radford, Tanya, *A Guide for Caregivers*, New York: National Multiple Sclerosis Society 1999.

Ratner, Rochelle, "But You Look So Good!," New York: National Multiple Sclerosis Society 1999.

Reingold, Stephen C., Ph.D., *Research Directions in Multiple Sclerosis*, New York: National Multiple Sclerosis Society 2000.

Roessler, Richard T., Ph.D. and Phillip Rumrill, Ph.D., *The Win-Win Approach to Reasonable Accommodations*, New York: National Multiple Sclerosis Society 1998.

Rolak, Loren A., M.D., *MS: An Historical Perspective*, New York: National Multiple Sclerosis Society 1996.

Sanford, Mary Eve, Ph.D., and Jack H. Petajan, M.D., *Multiple Sclerosis and Your Emotions*, New York: National Multiple Sclerosis Society 1999.

Sarnoff, Jane, and Denise M. Rector, R.D., *Food for Thought: MS and Nutrition*, New York: National Multiple Sclerosis Society 1998.

Schapiro, Randall T., M.D., "Medications Used in the Treatment of Multiple Sclerosis," *Physical Medicine Rehabilitation Clinic of North America*, May 1999, Vol. 10, No. 2.

Schapiro, Randall T., M.D., *Symptom Management in Multiple Sclerosis, 3rd Edition*, New York: Demos Medical Publishing, Co., Inc. 1998.

Schwarz, Shelley Peterman, *300 Tips for Making Life with Multiple Sclerosis Easier*, New York; Demos Publishing, Inc. 1999.

Senelick, Richard C., M.D., and Karla Dougherty, *Beyond Please and Thank You: The Disability Awareness Handbook for Families*, Co-Workers, and Friends, Birmingham, AL: HealthSouth Press 2001.

Senelick, Richard C., M.D., and Karla Dougherty, *Living with Stroke: A Guide for Families, 3rd Edition*, Birmingham, AL: HealthSouth Press 2001.

Senelick, Richard C., M.D., and Karla Dougherty, *Living with Brain Injury: A Guide for Families, 2nd Edition*, Birmingham, AL: HealthSouth Press 2001.

Solari, A., M.D., G. Filippini, M.D., P. Gasco, M.D., L. Colla, M.D., A. Salmaggi, M.D., L. La Mantia, M.D., M. Farinotti, M. Eoili, M.D., and L. Mendozzi, M.D., "Physical Rehabiltation has a Positive Effect on Disability in Multiple Sclerosis Patients," *Neurology* 1999, Vol. 52, No. 57.

Van Den Noort, Stanley, M.D., and Nancy J. Holland, Ed.D., *Multiple Sclerosis in Clinical Practice*, New York: Demos Medical Publishing, Inc. 1999.

Thompson, A.J., "Multiple Sclerosis: Rehabilitation Measures," *Seminars in Neurology*, 1998, Vol. 18, No. 3.

White, A.T., T.E. Wilson, and J.H. Petajan, "Effect of Pre-exercise Cooling on Physical Function and Fatigue in Multiple Sclerosis Patients, *Medical Science and Sports Exercise*, 1997, Vol. 29, Supplement 5.

INDEX

ABOUT THE AUTHOR

Richard C. Senelick, MD, is the medical director at HealthSouth Rehabilitation Institute of San Antonio (RIOSA). A native of Illinois, Dr. Senelick completed his undergraduate and medical school training at the University of Illinois in Chicago. A neurologist who specializes in neurorehabilitation, he subsequently completed his neurology training at the University of Utah in Salt Lake City. In addition to lecturing on both a National and International level, Dr. Senelick has authored numerous publications, including co-authoring *Living with Brain Injury: A Guide for Families*, *The Spinal Cord Injury Handbook for Patients and Their Families*, and *Living with Stroke: A Guide for Families*. Dr. Senelick is also editor-in-chief of HealthSouth Press.

"Getting People Back"
　　— The HEALTHSOUTH Rehabilitation Series

Getting people back . . . to work . . . to play . . . to living. It has been the HealthSouth commitment since we first started taking care of people with disabilities and injuries. Now HealthSouth Press continues this tradition with "Getting People Back"—The HealthSouth Rehabilitation Series.

These books are specifically designed for people who need up to date, authoritative and easy-to-access knowledge about their conditions. In a user friendly, simple manner, these books help educate patients and their families.

Through knowledge and education comes empowerment and the ability to do more than just "live" with disabling symptoms. These books provide the opportunity to exceed expectations and get people back.